TOP DOCTORS
Share Amazing
Stories Why You Need

CHELATION
THERAPY

and Other Vital

DETOX Methods to

SAVE YOUR LIFE

Published by Advantage, Charleston, South Carolina.
Member of Advantage Media Group.

ADVANTAGE is a registered trademark and the Advantage colophon is a trademark of Advantage Media Group, Inc.

Printed in the United States of America.

ISBN: 978-159932-571-2
LCCN: 2015935787

This publication is designed to provide accurate and authoritative information in regard to the subject matter covered. It is sold with the understanding that the publisher is not engaged in rendering legal, accounting, or other professional services. If legal advice or other expert assistance is required, the services of a competent professional person should be sought.

Advantage Media Group is proud to be a part of the Tree Neutral® program. Tree Neutral offsets the number of trees consumed in the production and printing of this book by taking proactive steps such as planting trees in direct proportion to the number of trees used to print books. To learn more about Tree Neutral, please visit **www.treeneutral.com**. To learn more about Advantage's commitment to being a responsible steward of the environment, please visit **www.advantagefamily.com/green**

Advantage Media Group is a publisher of business, self-improvement, and professional development books and online learning. We help entrepreneurs, business leaders, and professionals share their Stories, Passion, and Knowledge to help others Learn & Grow. Do you have a manuscript or book idea that you would like us to consider for publishing? Please visit **advantagefamily.com** or call **1.866.775.1696.**

TOP DOCTORS
Share Amazing
Stories Why You Need

CHELATION THERAPY

and Other Vital
DETOX Methods to
SAVE YOUR LIFE

Interviews by

Edward C. Kondrot, MD

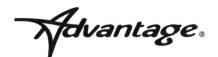

Dedicated to the brave pioneers in alternative medicine who are helping to restore health.

ACKNOWLEDGMENT

I want to thank all the doctors who have contributed to this book. They are located around the country; most have a national, if not international practice, and serve patients both locally and from afar. The stories of how and why they developed an interest in chelation and detox methods after undergoing training in conventional medicine or dentistry are almost as compelling as their discussions of techniques and modalities. On behalf of patients everywhere, I am especially grateful to these creative and selfless practitioners for affirming that "There is always hope, regardless of your pain or your diagnosis." Unfortunately, we often need to look beyond the limits of conventional medicine to hear this message. Fortunately, we now know where to look.

I extend thanks to Gloria St John for her major contribution in editing this book. As a practicing homeopath and medical researcher and editor, she brings a mix of talents that made the chapters in this book consistent and easy to understand for every type of reader. My cousin Christine Kondrot provided the final copyediting; I can always trust her sharp eye to produce an impeccable manuscript that reflects the intent of the authors.

Special thanks to Advantage Publishing for accomplishing the task of putting the printed material into book form.

Lastly, my greatest appreciation goes to my wonderful wife, Ly, who supported me in this important project.

Edward C. Kondrot, MD, MD(H), CCH, DHt

FOREWORD

by Garry Gordon, MD, DO

Co-Founder of the American College for Advancement in Medicine (ACAM)

You were meant to pick up this book! Your life is going to change dramatically for the better after you read it. What you have been told about heart disease and stroke—"take statins and eat a low-fat diet"—is nonsense. So is the information you have received about the cause and treatment of many other diseases. Learn how to avoid the medical morass of drugs, bypass surgery, stents, and even amputations of gangrenous legs. If you feel fatigued, you may have low level lead toxicity, and this book shows how to achieve a much better state of health.

The word "chelation" comes from the Greek word "claw" because a chelating agent is able to grab hold of a single atom of lead or mercury and safely remove it from the body. Because chelation therapy saved my life, I have made it my life's work to understand it, foster it, and help train other doctors to use it. The top chelation doctors who have contributed to this book have the good fortune to see miracles in their practices occurring all the time.

Many integrative physicians have been using chelation for decades, originally to treat heart disease, because we recognized it helps blood flow throughout the entire body. We used to think chelation worked like a roto-rooter, scrubbing the arteries of calcium buildup and thereby widening them. We now know chelation works primarily by lowering the body's load of heavy metal toxins which gum up the works in numerous ways. Heavy metals impair the ability of blood vessels to repair themselves. After chelation, blood vessels become younger and more flexible, like a new hose, not an old stiff one.

How does chelation therapy do that? It neutralizes the adverse effects of toxic heavy metals that are so prevalent now in our world and have found their way into us. We can't see, touch, or feel heavy metals. Sometimes they are hard to measure, but they are in our bones, our tissues, and our blood, and they exact a toll on our health every day.

Let's zero in on lead. Lead impairs mitochondrial function. The mitochondria are like the engine in a car—they are where the air we breathe and the food we eat gets turned into energy inside each of our 80 trillion or so cells. Each step required to make that energy is enzyme dependent. The enzymes require zinc and other minerals to make those conversions; *lead competes with zinc and other essential minerals*. Remove the lead—improve your metabolic function.

Chelation therapy came into wide use 40 years ago because of its demonstrated ability to improve blood flow throughout the entire body, which helps prevent heart attacks, strokes, and gangrene. Now, it is becoming clear that its potential applications are far broader than that. Chelation is also possibly the best way to improve kidney function and could make dialysis obsolete.

The TACT (Trial to Assess Chelation Therapy) study turned up something most of us had not zeroed in on before: chelation helps prevent death from diabetes. Diabetes is not just a disease of too much sugar. The mineral zinc is crucial to the functioning of the hormone insulin, which shuttles sugar out of the bloodstream. Lead, on the other hand, prevents zinc from doing its job. The higher the level of lead in the human body, the more poisonous sugar is because zinc and its associated enzymes cannot do their job. So the body calls for more and more insulin to drive corrosive sugar out of the bloodstream. The more sugar in the bloodstream, the more inflammation in the arteries, and the more the arteries thicken. If the situation gets bad enough, the extremities are starved for blood; your kidneys can stop working, your brain can be impaired, or your feet can become gangrenous—some part of the body is going to pay the price. With one-third of Americans overweight or obese, meaning they are pre-diabetic or diabetic, this has the makings of a treatment that can change many people's lives for the better.

Chelation could also have a significant impact on fatty liver disease—and every form of liver disease for that matter. Many of the symptoms of menopause are also caused by lead toxicity when the bone turnover may be so accelerated that a woman develops high blood pressure. Chelation therapy needs to become widely recognized as a vital step that helps many other major medical therapies work better, including pharmaceutical treatment for depression and cancer.

Heavy metals are also linked to autoimmune diseases, neurological problems, and even cancer. Improved blood flow in persons treated with chelation also led to better vision and memory, even improved sex lives. Finally, chelation therapy is the most effective anti-aging medicine available since it prevents premature death from the most common causes while increasing energy and vitality. In fact, our patients seem to become younger the more chelation they have.

So why is it so little known? Its potential to reduce surgical intervention and drug use threatens our medical institutions and the profitable treatments offered by hospitals and pharmaceutical companies. While the original focus of chelation therapy was on improving blood flow, practitioners soon determined that motivated patients could almost always return to an active life with no need for bypass surgery, stents, or other costly interventions.

Those of us who do chelation debate which therapy is best for which patient—the IV or the oral? Some patients are in for prevention; others are scheduled next week for amputation, so we need to be flexible in our approach. As you read through the chapters of this book, you will see that each doctor has developed an approach that produces the best results for their patients. You will also note that they are all interested in learning new techniques. This keeps the science and art of chelation therapy vital.

How does lead poison us? First of all, you need to know that lead is stored in the bones. Then, as the bone remodels—absorbing bone tissue and simultaneously depositing new bone—it releases a little lead which poisons all the other tissues of the body and sabotages the ability of enzymes to perform the millions of jobs they do daily to keep us alive. Even if we lived in a perfectly clean world with no lead in our water, food, or air from this day forward, we would still be at the mercy of the lead stored in our bones from birth which will continue to be released slowly for the rest of our lives.

In the 1970s, chelation therapy was gradually being undertaken by more and more primary care practitioners in spite of the threat from organized medicine and medical boards. By 1976, I had studied most of the research papers available on the topic, pulled that information together, and published it in *Osteopathic Annals* with a long list references. It is interesting to look back at that article today and see the editors' comments. Here are two of them:

"Vested interests will feel threatened by chelation therapy."

"The beneficial effect of chelation in chronic diseases is noteworthy."

Those vested interests are still very much at work 40 years later. Chelation therapy is the way we could eliminate 90 percent, or more, of vascular surgery including stents and bypasses. Could it be that the American medical establishment is over-utilizing these invasive procedures with associated risks including death, and under-utilizing a proven, safe, relatively inexpensive option like chelation therapy that has five decades of experience?

We estimate that 20 million people have received some form of chelation therapy. Currently, in the United States, there are perhaps 5,000 doctors who offer chelation. I hope many more doctors will choose to offer this therapy which, although not yet considered Standard of Care, dramatically changes the health of nearly every patient who undergoes chelation. Therapies that help the body remove or neutralize toxins must be a key part of any effective treatment program for any condition because our bodies simply were not designed to cope with the amount of lead, mercury, and other contaminants in our environment.

I congratulate Dr. Kondrot for publishing this compelling account of chelation in our country today as told by the leaders in the field. It is our hope that many who read this book will seek chelation to improve their already good health or to address chronic and life-threatening conditions. Lead—if you don't keep pushing it out, it is going to keep killing you.

TABLE OF CONTENTS

INTRODUCTION

When I first began writing and publishing books about natural medicine, I limited my topics to the wonderful results I had reversing eye disease, since I am an ophthalmologist. As I delved more deeply into natural healing methods, I soon discovered that things are a lot simpler than the world of specialized medicine would have you believe. In many cases of chronic illness, including eye disease, the underlying cause of the disorders is very simple—heavy metal poisoning. This one disease affects all of us on the planet to some degree and can be cured by getting the lead, mercury, and other toxins out of our bodies, bones, and brains.

The process of removing heavy metals is called chelation therapy and was introduced in the United States for removing lead in the 1950s. It has been officially limited to this application, although all doctors involved in this field have known for a long time that it has wider application, especially in the realm of cardiovascular diseases. Finally, in 2012, the results of the first federally funded large scale, longitudinal, double-blind, placebo-controlled study, the TACT (Trial to Assess Chelation Therapy), demonstrated chelation's remarkable effectiveness in reducing mortality in heart attack patients, especially in diabetic heart patients. While it is too soon to see how this information will affect treatment for circulatory disorders, the many pioneering practitioners of chelation and their patients are waiting for this development.

We are on the brink of a medical revolution on a par
with the discovery of penicillin.

Many of my colleagues asked me to bring the latest and now greatest news about chelation to the public as well as to the medical community at large. I interviewed a number of doctors who provide chelation treatment and asked them to describe their approach as well as their clinical results. Voila—this book—a compendium of chelation protocols, products, and spectacular cases. We will celebrate the book's publication at the first Chelation Therapy Conference in Florida in Spring 2015. The public will be invited to learn about this remarkable, safe, effective therapy that virtually every person on the planet needs.

I know you will want to investigate chelation as a possible treatment for yourself or someone you know after reading this book. I have published the list of organizations that set the standards for chelation as well as train doctors in this method. I encourage you to locate a doctor in your area, using the referral lists provided by the organizations below, and see if you can be the next miracle case!

Edward Kondrot, MD
Healing the Eye and Wellness Center
Dade City, Florida

RESOURCES
How to Find a Doctor or Dentist Trained in Detoxification Methods

Physicians

Academy of Comprehensive Integrative Medicine
www.academyofintegrativemedicine.com
866-308-9737

American Academy of Environmental Medicine
www.aaemonlilne.org
316- 684-5500

American Board of Clinical Metal Toxicology
www.abcmt.org
513-942-3226

American College for Advancement in Medicine

www.acam.org

1.800.LEADOUT

International College of Integrative Medicine

www.icimed.com

419-358-0273

Dentists

Holistic Dental Association

www.holisticdental.org

305-356-7338

International Academy of Biological Dentistry and Medicine

www.iabdm.org

281-651-1745

International Academy of Oral Medicine and Toxicology

www.iaomt.org

863-420-6373

CHELATION: THE KEY TO A LONG AND HEALTHY LIFE

Interview with
Terry Chappell, MD

Dr. Chappell graduated from the University of Michigan Medical School in 1969. He is certified in Family Practice, Geriatrics, Chelation Therapy, Pain Management, and Advanced Longevity Medicine. As past president of the International College of Integrative Medicine, past president of the American College for Advancement in Medicine, and as a volunteer assistant clinical professor of medicine at Wright State College of Medicine, he has taught chelation therapy and other integrative subjects to students and to doctors around the world. He has published widely on chelation therapy in scientific journals and in popular books. He has served as a consultant for National Institutes of Health on several occasions. He is in private practice with the Celebration of Health Association in Bluffton and Toledo, Ohio.

Dr. Chappell became interested in alternatives after becoming frustrated with the results and complications he was seeing with conventional drugs and surgery. He now devotes his practice to safe, natural techniques to improve function and help the body heal. He has assembled a high team to get the best results possible with each patient. They offer many innovative therapies for pain relief, allergy desensitization, circulation improvement, energy enhancement, hormone balancing, and joint stabilization.

1. **When results from the chelation study were presented, it was clear that the patients who received chelation therapy did significantly better than the ones who did not.**

2. **If you want to live not only a long life but also a healthy life, and one that is free from disability and dependency, you need to keep your arteries in shape. There's nothing better than chelation therapy to do that.**

3. **As soon as he started the therapy, he started feeling better. During the next three years, he was not admitted to the coronary care unit even once as opposed to spending one third of his life there before treatment.**

. . . .

Dr. Kondrot: Please tell us a bit about your medical training and how you became interested in chelation and detoxification.

Dr. Chappell: I went to medical school at the University of Michigan and graduated in 1969. I completed a rotating internship in Utah, and then I practiced for a year in Harlan, Kentucky. Our clinic was affiliated with the University of Kentucky.

Eventually, I sat for my board exams and became certified in family practice. Since then, I've been recertified six or seven times. I was very interested in family medicine. At the time I became certified, there was a big push toward more prevention in medicine. Paying attention to exercise, diet, and minimizing the effects of stress and coping with it effectively were all essential parts of the program.

After beginning my practice in Appalachia, I moved to Bluffton, Ohio, where I still live. There were a lot of people in Appalachia who were underprivileged. Many were on Medicaid. It seemed like most had prescriptions for pain pills and antidepressants just to cope with the problems they had in their lives. It's not that they wanted it, but that was the only treatment offered to them.

I thought there had to be a better way, so I looked for alternative treatments that might work instead. My wife, a registered nurse, inspired me by teaching Lamaze natural childbirth classes. I found a couple of treatments that were very effective. I started with hypnosis and then learned auriculotherapy, a form of ear acupuncture that is commonly used in France. My patients responded very well, and I became excited by alternative medicine as opposed to drugs and surgery. As I attended more meetings and learned how to apply alternative treatments, I began to see the importance of detoxification.

A few years later, one of my patients was the CEO of a company that had several employees who had benefited from chelation. They drove all the way from northwestern Ohio to West Virginia to get their treatments. He urged me to look into providing chelation in my practice. I was still fairly fresh out of medical school, and I thought I knew more than I actually did, so I was pretty skeptical about it initially. He eventually convinced me to visit a couple of doctors who were doing chelation therapy. I was astounded at how effective the treatment seemed to be. By talking to the patients, I learned that many of them had a history of severe illness. Chelation helps with detoxification of heavy metals, such as lead, mercury, and arsenic, and also tends to improve circulation throughout the body. They were now functioning well and living a virtually normal life. I said to myself, "I'm going to have to look into this."

I went to a workshop to learn how to provide the therapy through the American Association of Medical Preventics (later called the American College for the Advancement of Medicine—ACAM). I not only learned how to provide the therapy to my patients, but I eventually became president of the organization. Since then, I've also served five terms as president of the International College of Integrative Medicine—ICIM, and I've been involved in teaching chelation to doctors for many years. It's been a wonderful and gratifying experience.

. . . .

Dr. Kondrot: You were involved with the landmark Trial to Assess Chelation Therapy, or the TACT study. That was certainly very exciting for all doctors who believed in chelation to have a national study that was supervised by the federal government. Please tell us about your role in that study and the results.

Dr. Chappell: When I was first involved with ACAM, the AMA challenged the chelation doctors to do a study. The AMA's contention was if they're going to promote a therapy, they ought to perform research on it. The only trouble was that the physicians in ACAM were not research doctors, so they had to pair up with a medical school or some research center. Several attempts at doing that were unsuccessful, but finally the National Institutes of Health responded to a hearing held by Congress. Representative Dan Burton of Indianapolis presided over the hearing. The National Institutes of Health then funded a study on chelation therapy that began around 2000. I was involved because they asked me sit on the panels to evaluate the applications to perform the study.

Eventually, the study proposed by Dr. Gervasio (Tony) Lamas was chosen to be funded. Tony is a renowned research cardiologist from Florida. There were 134 sites in the study from around the country with a few from Canada. Some were medical schools and others were experienced chelating physicians. Patients were followed for five years.

Everyone in the study needed to have had a heart attack, and they had to continue evidence-based conventional medical care.

There were four groups:

- Chelation and high dose vitamins (best results)
- Chelation and low dose vitamins (good results)
- Placebo and high dose vitamins (no statistical improvement)
- Double placebo/no treatment (no statistical improvement)

The study was completed in 2011. It took longer than we thought. It was difficult to get patients enrolled because the cardiology community wasn't enthusiastic about it and actually discouraged patients from participating. There were 1,708 patients enrolled. The results were first presented at a national meeting of the American Heart Association.

When Dr. Lamas presented the data, it was clear that the patients who received chelation therapy did significantly better than the ones who did not. As the results were presented to a huge room full of practicing cardiologists from around the country, you could hear a pin drop. It was exactly the opposite of what they expected.

At a subsequent meeting of the American Heart Association, the details of the study were presented. The biggest improvement occurred in patients who were diabetic. As it turned out, in this five-year period, the patients who were diabetic and received chelation therapy plus high-dose vitamins had 51 percent fewer cardiac events than the patients who were given placebos. This is an incredible result that shows EDTA (ethylenediaminetetraacetic acid) chelation plus high-dose multivitamins to be more effective than most medications that are approved by the FDA. For example, a study presented at a recent AHA meeting showed that adding Vytorin to a statin drug reduced future cardiac events by six percent over seven years. This result generated spectacular headlines in the news media.

Since that time, Dr. Lamas has presented the TACT study results at many medical schools and to the National Institutes of Health and the FDA. All were impressed. The problem is that the FDA doesn't usually approve a treatment on the basis of one study. They insisted that we have a second study.

In the early fall of 2014, Dr. Lamas announced that he was going to proceed with a second major study for chelation therapy. The first one was called TACT, the Trial to Assess Chelation Therapy. The second one is called TACT 2. It will enroll diabetic patients who have had a heart attack and follow them for three years instead of five. If it comes out the way the first one did, which is certainly expected, chelation will hopefully become a routine treatment for vascular disease.

. . . .

Dr. Kondrot: To make it clear, there were favorable results not only in the diabetic group but also the other group of individuals who had a history of heart disease. I wonder if you could talk a little bit about the statistics in that group.

Dr. Chappell: The overall statistics showed a reduction in cardiac events of 18 percent in the chelation group that did not receive high-dose vitamins. The reduction was 26 percent when high-dose vitamins were added. Diabetics showed the best results. Diabetes is a vascular disease. The complications are vascular problems. There was a statistically significant improvement for patients in the TACT study who had chelation therapy. The results confirm the experience of doctors who use chelation therapy. However, the results are even more impressive in the smaller studies that have been performed by those doctors who routinely provide chelation, including myself. We expected an even greater improvement than was found in the formal study.

That's often the case when you conduct such a study. There are a lot of factors to be considered. For example, patients treated in the office usually continue to receive monthly maintenance treatments after the basic course of 30 weekly IVs. TACT patients were treated for only 18 months but were followed for five years. Furthermore, doctors who provide chelation therapy almost always add additional nutritional therapies as needed, which was not part of the TACT protocol. The study confirmed the overall impression that we had, although I think we can do a lot better for patients in clinical practice than was apparent in the study.

Dr. Kondrot: Finally there's a study that supports clinically what many of us have observed for the last decade. What can you tell the public about the key points they need to know about chelation?

Dr. Chappell: Chelation therapy is a dynamic therapy that has at least two major effects. One is that it detoxifies heavy metals. Three out of the top four toxic substances in the United States are toxic metals. Those are arsenic, lead, and mercury. EDTA chelation therapy removes all of those metals, although sometimes an additional chelating substance might be used to remove mercury. In addition, EDTA improves circulation all over the body. The number-one cause of death is heart disease, and stroke is not far behind. Many other diseases like diabetes have circulation problems as a component. Common eye disorders such as macular degeneration and glaucoma are caused by circulation problems.

EDTA chelation is the only therapy we have that can address both of these mechanisms, so it's a powerful therapy that should have a huge impact on extending life and improving the quality of life in people as they get older. It is beautiful as a longevity medicine because it reduces the chance of having a heart attack or a stroke, which are leading causes of death and disability.

Dr. Kondrot: Please give an example of life-changing events that you have noticed with patients in your practice.

Dr. Chappell: One of the most dramatic cases was a gentleman who came to me when he was about 60 years of age. He had spent one third of his life and the previous three years in the cardiac care unit. In other words, he was an inpatient in the hospital in the unit that cares for patients with severe cardiac problems. When he was discharged from the hospital, he couldn't function. He couldn't do anything but walk slowly around the house. He was an invalid.

He came to me and wanted chelation therapy. I began treatments. The amazing thing was that as soon as he started the therapy, he started feeling better. During the next three years, he was not admitted to the coronary care unit even once as opposed to one third of his life before treatment. He started bowling again. He resumed playing golf. He had not been able to do those things for years. He felt much better and had a dramatic improvement in the quality of his life. Despite my admonitions, he continued to smoke for the three years during the time he was treated. That was something that should have made him worse, but it didn't.

That could be the most dramatic case I've had, but we've had quite a few similar cases. In fact, if you visit a doctor who does chelation therapy and talk to the patients who are receiving it, you'll hear amazing results. Many are people who have had multiple cardiac surgeries, heart attacks, strokes, or were labeled "cardiac cripples." Many are now normal. Chelation is not 100 percent successful, but it is an excellent therapy.

Dr. Kondrot: Have you undergone chelation therapy? I met you personally, and you have a lot of energy and are very youthful.

Dr. Chappell: Thank you. Yes, I have. As a matter of fact, just recently I finished my 300th treatment. As I said, the usual basic course of therapy is weekly treatments for 30 weeks. Often, people will elect to continue to take maintenance treatments about once a month. Over the years, my 300 treatments have averaged to about ten treatments a year. I developed some angina symptoms in the 1980s.

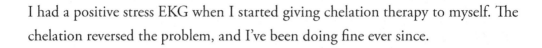

I had a positive stress EKG when I started giving chelation therapy to myself. The chelation reversed the problem, and I've been doing fine ever since.

. . . .

Dr. Kondrot: Many conventional doctors are prescribing treatments they would never consider for themselves. How about the safety issue of chelation therapy?

Dr. Chappell: There's minimal risk involved. You have to be careful to monitor kidney function. If you give too much chelation too fast, you could put a little strain on the kidneys. For that reason, we're very cautious when we give chelation. We individualize the dose, based on the patient's kidney function. There are studies published in the *Journal of American Medical Association* and elsewhere that show that EDTA chelation therapy can actually improve the status of patients with mild to moderate kidney failure. You just have to be very careful not to overload the kidneys when removing toxic metals.

Chelation is a very safe treatment. Other side effects are rare and easy to treat. As a matter of fact, part of the TACT study on chelation therapy looked at safety factors, and they didn't find any problems at all. That's important because chelation has been criticized in the past for being a dangerous therapy, but that did not show up at all when it was studied carefully.

. . . .

Dr. Kondrot: That's remarkable. Something as common as taking an aspirin tablet has known complications such as hemorrhages and other problems. Absolutely no side effects or complications were reported in the chelation study.

Dr. Chappell: That's right. It's out of the ordinary. Medications usually have side effects. Of course, the patients in the study aged five to seven years, so some usual symptoms of aging were noted. But there were actually a few more problems in the placebo group than in the chelation group.

. . . .

Dr. Kondrot: The public is often confused by the various methods that are marketed for chelation therapy. Please describe some of your favorite ways to detoxify.

Dr. Chappell: Over the years, there has been considerable research that's been done on chelation therapy. I've published some of the papers myself. Most of the studies were not double-blind and did not have placebo controls. They're not sufficient to present to the FDA for general acceptance, but they certainly do confirm the results of the therapy.

One of the problems we face is that companies have manufactured and promoted oral medicines and herbal products that are called chelators that are supposedly effective for removing toxic metals. Typically, these companies quote the research that has been done on intravenous chelation therapy and make a claim that the oral preparations are just as effective. They are definitely not as effective. I give EDTA chelation therapy intravenously as a powerful detoxification program.

However, if somebody uses an oral chelator to prevent absorption of toxins from the food supply, it might be useful. Only about five percent of EDTA is absorbed into the body when taken by mouth. Oral EDTA is not sufficient to lower the body's burden of toxic metals, but it might help prevent further accumulation.

Exercise is very important as well. Sauna therapy can be helpful. For removing toxic chemicals other than heavy metals, some herbal products are effective, including milk thistle. We use that quite a bit. Colonic irrigation and high-fiber supplements are good detoxifying measures.

. . . .

Dr. Kondrot: How do you evaluate patients before chelation therapy to see if they're good candidates, and what parameters do you use to monitor their success with chelation?

Dr. Chappell: In our office, we sometimes call it the triple play when we're evaluating for patients who might need chelation therapy or improvement in circulation. We do a test for toxic metals. Most toxic metals only stay in the bloodstream for a week or two when they come into the body. Then they're stored in the bone, brain, or fat tissue. If you rely on a blood test, you're only going to get what the recent exposure is. You're not going to determine what patients have had as a lifetime accumulation of toxic metals.

First, we do a urine challenge test by giving a dose of EDTA, sometimes with DMSA. We then measure the urine to determine the load of toxic metals the patient has. The second test we use is a max pulse test, which is a heart rate variability test with analysis of the pulse wave. That tells us how the heart is functioning, particularly under stress. This is a tool that is often used to see how much damage stress is causing on the heart. The third test we do in the office is a carotid artery ultrasound, which measures the intimal thickness and plaque development of the carotid arteries. If there's plaque or thickness in that artery, vascular disease is developing.

Usually, we perform all three of these tests. Of course, we also look at standard heart and circulation tests that are often performed in the hospital. Included might be stress EKGs, Doppler testing, ultrasounds, CT scans, and catheterizations. All of these tests give added information, but we are careful to minimize the cost whenever possible.

Our triple play can be repeated during the treatment to see if patients are getting better or worse. In the case of chelation therapy, they almost always get better. Some of the studies I was involved with showed a pretty consistent improvement rate of 87 to 90 percent with measurable testing after they received chelation therapy.

. . . .

Dr. Kondrot: After you evaluate someone and you feel he or she is a good candidate for chelation, what is the protocol you use?

Dr. Chappell: We plan out a series of treatments. If all they have is toxic metals—and this may happen in a younger person—they may need only ten intravenous treatments. Then we repeat the challenge test to see if another course of therapy is needed.

If there's a vascular problem, the basic course of treatment is 30 treatments. In our office, we usually do them once a week. We assess their kidney function and monitor it to see if there's any strain on the kidneys. If there is, we reduce the dose and spread out the treatments. We encourage an ample intake of water. That enables us to give the treatment safely.

There are a lot of adjuncts you can use with chelation therapy. Exercise is probably the most powerful lifestyle factor you can do to treat vascular problems and prevent heart attacks. We always talk about a healthy diet, which includes mostly fresh fruits and vegetables and foods that are good, clean, and nutritious.

We also want to see how patients are dealing with stress. Most patients in today's world have stress in their lives, and that can be very detrimental if it gets to be excessive.

We check vitamin D levels. Vitamin D has been linked to vascular disease as well as cancer and osteoporosis. Homocysteine, ferritin, and C-reactive protein blood levels can also be important.

We add other supplements if patients have other symptoms. We can often improve their cardiac function by using D-ribose, L-carnitine, Coenzyme Q10, magnesium, Hawthorne berry, and taurine. I like nattokinase and natural vitamin E to decrease excessive clotting.

We want to control their blood pressure. If their cholesterol is excessively high, we will improve that as well. Usually we can accomplish both with natural therapies. Cinnamon, berberine, and red yeast can often do a very effective job with lipids and glucose control. Magnesium and herbal products can lower the blood pressure. Garlic and Rauwolfia can be effective without the side effects of many anti-hypertensive medicines.

Sometimes we look at amino acids, particularly L-arginine, which can improve nitric oxide production, which dilates the blood vessels. Lysine shouldn't be taken at the same time of day as L-arginine, but a combination of vitamin C and lysine can help reduce lipoprotein (a), which is one of the most potent risk factors in the blood.

There are many things we can do to enhance the results of treatment. We don't want to rely just on chelation therapy. It's an excellent therapy, but it's not perfect, and there are a lot of other things you can do to help it along.

. . . .

Dr. Kondrot: Please share a patient story that relates to heavy metal toxicity, presenting symptoms, and how chelation helped that individual.

Dr. Chappell: Heavy metals can cause a lot of problems. Many of the problems are not obviously related to the metals. They occur under the surface, and they can help cause chronic degenerative diseases such as heart attacks, strokes, cancer, and autoimmune problems.

There are several specific connections of toxic metals to diseases. Mercury is one. Many years ago in the beginning of this country, people sought beaver pelts so they could make luxurious hats, which were very popular in Europe. However, the process of making those hats involved using mercury. The people who made the hats were known later as "mad hatters" because the mercury they used caused them to have severe mental problems. They became so toxic that they often died at a younger age. As we remove mercury from the body today, we notice less in the way of anxiety, depression, and memory problems.

Interestingly enough, one of the symptoms I have noticed with lead toxicity is in the digestive tract. Many patients with toxic metals have digestive problems such as constipation, diarrhea, gas, or bloating. Such symptoms often improve as you remove lead from the body. Many toxic metals have symptoms of chronic degenerative diseases such as pain in the joints, headaches, and fatigue. They often improve as you reduce the toxic load of metals.

. . . .

Dr. Kondrot: If an individual has really bad veins or they don't want to do IV chelation, do you have a particular protocol you recommend to help them?

Dr. Chappell: A lot of supplements I mentioned before help with circulation in general. For veins, I often recommend horse chestnut.

Plaque in the arteries often leaks a little fatty material, and the body responds to that by forming a clot around the fatty material. That can break off, go downstream, and block off the artery. As a matter of fact, that is the mechanism for probably 80 percent of heart attacks and strokes. Anything you can do to modify this process is helpful.

Oxidized LDL cholesterol plays a role in the process. Inflammation also plays a significant role, in my opinion. You can reduce inflammation in the vascular tree with enzymes and various herbal preparations that also quiet inflammation in the joints. A natural statin like red yeast is also helpful. Nattokinase is a favorite of mine because it helps prevent the clotting response to plaque leakage. It also helps reduce inflammation.

. . . .

Dr. Kondrot: Please share some key takeaway points that you feel are essential for patients reading this.

Dr. Chappell: One takeaway point is that the first sign of a heart attack or stroke can be sudden death. Hypertension is sometimes called the silent killer because you don't necessarily have obvious symptoms of vascular problems before it hits you like a sledgehammer.

I think it's very important that people live a healthy lifestyle, deal with stress, eat a good diet, and get regular exercise. Those are the cornerstones of effective preventive medicine.

You should do some test for vascular screening to see if you have early signs of circulation problems. Your doctor can recommend what would be best for you. Some of the tests we discussed today can be very useful.

If you want to live not only a long life but also a healthy life, and one that is free from disability and dependence on other people, you really need to keep your arteries in shape. There's nothing better than chelation therapy to do that. I'm absolutely convinced that chelation is a wonderful therapy that can help circulation all over the body. Chelation can help you function better for the rest of your life.

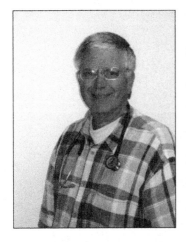

Terry Chappell, MD
Celebration of Health Association
122 Thurman Street, Box 248
Bluffton, OH 45817
800-788-4627
mail@healthcelebration.com
www.healthcelebration.com

DETOXIFY
THE NATURAL WAY

Interview with
Dennis Courtney, MD

Dr. Courtney brings his unique experiences to his patients through the many careers he enjoyed before entering the practice of medicine. No career better describes his contributions than "Teacher." His classroom is now his office, and his students are the patients who consult him about a myriad of problems

When his patients leave his office, they know that they have just initiated a relationship that is very unique. They also know they have found a knowledgeable advocate in their quest to achieve longevity with quality of life. The fact that they feel like they have just left a classroom suits Dr. Courtney just fine.

Dr. Courtney earned his medical degree from the University of Nuevo Leon in Monterrey, Mexico, and returned to Pittsburgh, Pennsylvania, to take up his specialty training in anesthesiology at West Penn Hospital. Upon completing his residency in 1986, he embarked on a medical practice, dividing his time between the operating room and his newfound interest in managing patients in chronic pain.

"The Courtney Medical Group" refers to a unique set of therapies that have advantages over the more conventional treatment approaches that they are meant to replace. In all cases, these treatment programs are non-toxic and do not rely upon pharmaceuti-

cals. They continue to evaluate new and promising treatment protocols as they become available, and the most promising therapies will be included in what they offer at "The Courtney Medical Group".

1. **The aging process always leads to the development of disorders, symptoms, and disease, and one of their root causes is an accumulation of toxic substances.**

2. **It becomes very difficult to justify using harsh (chelating) substances even to correct toxic issues.**

3. **My "three-legged stool" for healing is correct all deficiencies, remove all toxicities, and improve the blood flow to the organs.**

. . . .

Dr. Kondrot: Dr. Courtney, I am glad you are part of this exciting book. Please tell us a little bit about your medical training and how you became interested in chelation and detoxification.

Dr. Courtney: My medical training came at the end of a number of careers. Medicine is not my first love; it turned out to be my fifth. By the time medicine tapped me on the shoulder, I was 28 years old and I had to make a decision. To be medically trained, I had to go outside the country, so I entered medical school at the University of Nuevo León in Monterrey, Mexico. After completing those studies as well as the social service stint required by the Mexican government, I returned to the United States and entered an anesthesia residency at the West Penn Hospital in Pittsburgh, Pennsylvania.

After completion, I worked in the operating rooms of a number of hospitals in the western Pennsylvania area performing the typical duties of an anesthesiologist: preparing patients for surgery, allowing them to have surgery pain-free, and then emerging them from the anesthetic onto full recovery and discharge.

Soon, a gentleman began to mentor me in the use of alternative and integrative medicine. I really had no training for it at all as may be said for any doctor. Medical schools don't train you to think outside the box; you have to be mentored for that. My mentor's name was Dr. Arthur Cook. He's since deceased, but he provided me with an impetus to move into an arena that has continued to grow every day. Many years later, after a lot of due diligence and dedication, I now do the mentoring. This is how we pass it on.

. . . .

Dr. Kondrot: How did you become interested in chelation and detoxification?

Dr. Courtney: While I was working as an anesthesiologist, people began to tell me about things they were doing for themselves and their health that I had not heard about before. I said, "I don't know what you're talking about. Tell me more." One of the things that kept coming up was that they were undergoing something called chelation. I had never heard the word before. They were doing it for cardio-vascular benefit.

I said, "I'm a medical doctor. I've never heard about anything that can do what you describe. They said, "That's par for the course. You're a medical doctor. You'd be the last to know about this." Then they gave me information which led me to more information, some written by medical doctors for medical doctors.

Now I had a big dilemma. I began to see that there were other areas of medicine, pretty well-developed, that I had never heard about in my formal medical training. Not only did I not hear about it, but I also could not find any references to it no matter how painstakingly I scoured the literature. It just wasn't there. That was my first inkling that something sinister was going on.

Now, many years later, there's still not much written about these areas, but there certainly has been a lot of new information that has allowed me to move forward in other arenas, particularly in chelation therapy.

. . . .

Dr. Kondrot: Can you recall a specific event that motivated you to look at this in more detail? Maybe it was a patient or some type of clinical result.

Dr. Courtney: I was looking for more information, and finally I realized there was a way to be educated in chelation therapy. Within 90 days, I was taking a course on how to perform it. I was told by the instructors, "Go back home and use these EDTA procedures. You're going to see a lot of benefit with your own patients." I came back home and rather tepidly and timidly introduced this into my practice. Within a few weeks, I began to get subjective feedback from my patients on how good they were feeling. When the objective information began to come through, the studies that were done before and after chelation, I was elated. From that point, it just continued. Since then, chelation for cardiovascular conditions continues to be a big part of my practice.

. . . .

Dr. Kondrot: That's interesting that your patients motivated you to explore this area, and now you've become a leading expert. What is the important information that the public should know about chelation and detoxification?

Dr. Courtney: Some generalities can be stated. First, if you are ill or if you have disagreeable symptoms, it's almost certain that toxicities are playing a role in your disease or symptoms. It affects us all, whether it's recognized by medical professionals or not. I guarantee you that toxicity is playing a role in your disease process.

If you're healthy, you're healthy for one of two reasons. One is that you belong to a growing group of people who caught on early in their lives and planned how they wanted to live. They are diligent about what and how they eat. In those patients, health isn't happening by accident. It's happening by design. That's one group of people who remain healthy.

The other group is people who just haven't gone far enough yet to experience the effects of the toxicities that they are accruing. We normally don't see our young adults afflicted. They're the immortals. Nothing seems to attack them, get them down, or provoke symptoms until later in life.

I can assure you that the aging process always will lead to the presentation of disorders, symptoms, and disease. Whatever diseases manifest, they will have, as one of the root causes, an accumulation of toxic substances that have grown to the point that the body can no longer do any enzymatic workarounds. The first disagreeable symptoms will emerge, and those disagreeable symptoms will continue to accrue. Until the toxic element of that disease is dealt with, one can never really re-establish a state of health.

· ·

Dr. Kondrot: What is your unique approach to not only chelation but to evaluating the patient and beginning some type of program?

Dr. Courtney: As an alternative doctor, I rarely prescribe any drugs if they can be avoided. The truth is that they can almost always be avoided, so I don't use pharmaceutical agents. As a general rule, patients come to me because they want to be managed by someone who's not going to prescribe drugs.

Formerly, as a very enthusiastic chelation doctor and detoxifier, I was using some of the harshest and potentially most harmful substances known to the pharmaceutical world. There's EDTA, DMSA, and DMPS. Those letters stand for pretty long words. I don't even know half of what the letters stand for. It became very difficult to justify using these harsh substances even to correct toxic issues. It's like saying it's okay to use these pharmaceutical agents when, in fact, it really is not.

As I've grown and learned more, my patients demanded that I pursue and establish some level of integrity and purity about how we approach these things, and they encouraged me to look beyond the use of these substances. I'm glad they did. It turns out they're all avoidable too. I've found other, better, safer, healthier ways to get rid of heavy metal burdens and toxic loads.

· ·

Dr. Kondrot: I'm very interested in hearing about these other ways. The typical physician does use IV chelation. It's a series of treatments to remove heavy metals. Any time there's a different approach that may be safer or more economical, it's always of interest to everyone.

Dr. Courtney: It's possible that some of my colleagues are undergoing the same self-searching that I went through. The chelation that was used for the cardio-vascular conditions that were brought to me way back in the mid-1990s—EDTA chelation—is the only way I know to help remove plaque on the inside of arteries. If that's the challenge, I know of no other way to help it other than using one of those chemical substances. We've made it extremely safe.

Now, however, so many people are seeing me for reasons other than cardiovascular. They come to me with every type of disease known to man. They have to be relieved of their toxic load if they are going to be healthy again.

I have a set of hierarchical ways of dealing with toxicity that I'll share with you now. First, there are foods that are great detoxifiers in themselves. People don't really appreciate how important this can be. The list of foods is a long one. One that many people know about is cilantro, which is extremely good for heavy metals, particularly mercury. Some other foods that are great detoxifiers are almonds, beets, cranberries, garlic, and kale. The list goes on. When using diet to help alleviate a toxic burden, only organic food should be used.

A second detoxifier that is relatively new to my practice is the use of essential oils. These are extracts that come from plants or seeds of plants. They were, and, in some cultures still are, the first medicines used. They've had a recent resurgence, and they're on their way back. There are a couple of really good companies that put together many extracts that have medicinal benefit. One of those medicinal benefits is to be able to detoxify. Based on the formula, you can ingest these oils, put them on the skin topically, or diffuse them so they're aromatic and you inhale them. That is another powerful way to detoxify. My patients really enjoy using essential oils. They like to have a diffuser going on in their own homes, kitchens, bedrooms, and the like. It's a pleasant way of accomplishing a medical goal.

. . . .

Dr. Kondrot: I know you use microcurrent as another way of potentiating the effect of these oils and helping them as a carrier going into the skin. Can you tell us which oils seem to work, the dosages, and how to apply them? It's the same thing with the cilantro. How do you make it part of your diet, and how much do you take?

Dr. Courtney: In terms of the foods, many of these things can be put into a salad mixed with essential fats and oils. It can be very tasty. You eat the foods in the amount you desire. One doesn't have to get so much down in the weeds worrying about certain dosages of those foods.

When it comes to the essential oils, you can atomize them after diluting them in water. There are other devices that allow you to use the full-strength oils. These may be needed by someone who has a greater load.

I will take the opportunity to discuss one other unique way of detoxifying. That's an approach that I first learned about through Patricia Kane, PhD. Patricia's approach involves the use of lipids, in particular phosphatidylcholine, one of the primary phospholipids found in normal cell membranes. The lipids can literally super-saturate a cell and gain entrance into the cell that no other substance can achieve. You can use them intravenously or orally.

Once you gain access to the cell, a second substance called glutathione can be added to the cell. Whether it's used orally or intravenously, it turns out to be a great detoxifier. By the way, it's the body's own natural detoxifier. Patricia Kane's protocol, which we affectionately refer to as the PK protocol, plays a prominent role in my office.

This is keeping with the newer philosophies to steer clear of the toxic pharmaceuticals and move to completely natural substances that don't really have any side effects. They can detoxify and relieve people of heavy metal burdens even better than the toxic agents do.

The last one is microcurrent. I believe it to be the medicine of the future. As I learn more about microcurrent, I see that it can be used for literally any disease in any part of the body. Toxicity is one condition it can address. Microcurrent is an absolutely great way to alleviate the burden of heavy metals and other toxic substances.

Microcurrent, with emphasis on the micro, provides a new way to use current. Electrical currents have been used in medicine for 20 or 30 years, but, in the past, the current was very high. It was macrocurrent, not microcurrent. It was measured in milliamperes. This is a large gush of electricity that can't be harnessed very well.

Microcurrent uses electrical currents that have been stepped down to simulate the same electrical activity that moves through the body naturally and allows it to function and exist. We use microamperes, a millionth of an ampere. At that level, there's great medical benefit by being able to simulate the body's own natural movement of energy, put tissue that's not healthy in harmony with health, and put diseases that are very detrimental at odds with that harmony to restore health once again.

It gets so specific that we can encourage detoxification from nose to toes. We can literally pick a body part, focus on it, and allow only it to be treated with microcurrent. We can pick the pathologies that are related to the person's own personal history. They may have a heavy metal burden, but maybe they had a vaccine injury as a child, or an automobile accident that led to a concussion. All of these elements can be programmed into these miraculous units to optimize their detoxification program.

This is the medicine of the future. It is where things are heading. It's certainly heading that way in my office, and I know it's absolutely part of yours, Dr. Kondrot. I want to thank you for introducing me to it and allowing me to gain more knowledge about this wonderful treatment. I know you didn't invent microcurrent, but you certainly popularized it and demonstrated how effective it can be, specifically in treating eye diseases.

. . . .

Dr. Kondrot: Have you found that any of these treatments have a synergistic effect? By combining microcurrent with essential oils or maybe even combining microcurrent with an IV chelation, have you observed a synergistic effect?

Dr. Courtney: The sun should never rise and set on one particular therapy, especially when the therapies are non-toxic. The patient really benefits from the synergy of combining multiple therapies. One's diet can easily be augmented with aromatherapy in the home while still taking a generous dose of lipids, some in the diet. You can do all of these at the same time. With each added modality, the benefits to the patient get exponentially better.

Who knows what's around the corner? There will be newer approaches. Look how these emerged. Look where we are now. I'm using all of them at the same time. Why not? None of them harms the patient in any way. You raised the question, is synergy expected? It's absolutely expected, and patients really appreciate it.

Dr. Kondrot: Can you could give us an example of a patient you evaluated and treated where you used many or all of these modalities in order to achieve a successful outcome.

Dr. Courtney: I've worked with some pretty serious conditions. One comes to mind immediately. I had a patient who was suffering from ALS which is a terminal neurological disease where the nerve impulses are not carried properly, and, as a result, the muscles aren't innervated. As it progresses, the person gets very weak, can't speak, can't walk, and is wheelchair-confined. The condition is usually rapid in its progression. It leads to almost certain death. It's one of the most terrible diseases possible. It's also called Lou Gehrig's disease.

I consider a person with ALS to be a high-priority patient. Naturally, whenever they come in, we'll use everything we have to help them. When I first met this patient, she could not make intelligible sounds. She was in a wheelchair. She wasn't intubated and was still able to breathe on her own, but she was very advanced in the disease process.

We used combinations of everything we just mentioned. The diet was completely changed. It had to be ground up into a liquid form because she couldn't tolerate or swallow chunks of food. We used the lipid approach I mentioned. We were using phosphatidylcholine and glutathione, as I described in the PK protocol. We also brought in microcurrent. We could set the frequencies to deal with the muscular system, neuromuscular system, the brain, and the nerves themselves.

Within the first month, the woman was restored to walking and talking on the telephone again. I had never really had an ALS patient before, but I know—and the patient knew—that this improvement was the result of all the therapies that we were using.

What about the synergy? The synergy worked for a very serious disease in a woman who I'm not so sure had much longer to live had we not met. She's so memorable to me that the moment you asked me to talk about a particular patient, she came to mind. She's still doing rather well. She doesn't need too much IV anymore. She does most of the protocol orally. This can work in a disease where there is absolutely no hope. Conventional medicine offers no hope to someone with Lou Gehrig's disease or ALS. Within a month, we were able to get this woman turned around.

She's a shining example of how well alternative medicine can work. Evidently, the toxicity issue played a large role in her disease and was not recognized by anybody else, but it became a high priority for us. That's my answer whenever somebody asks me, "Do you have a patient in mind?" She's present in my mind all the time.

· ·

Dr. Kondrot: Can you review the actual modalities you used with this patient? Do you have a certain way to evaluate a patient you think is toxic? Do you begin with laboratory testing or energetic testing? What do you typically start them on? Is there a sequence you use?

Dr. Courtney: Whenever we work with neurological diseases, in particular, we use a special lab. The only place to get this work done is from the Kennedy Krieger Institute's Peroxisomal Diseases Laboratory at Johns Hopkins University. They can measure the red blood cell membrane content that Dr. Patricia Kane uses to determine how deranged the membranes are. The membrane turns out to be an important part of any disease, and certainly neurological diseases. The standard labs are also obtained, but this particular test is unique to Patricia Kane's approach. It's certainly how we start with somebody with a disease as serious as ALS.

We begin with that, and then modify the diet because we don't use drugs. There are no drugs that help with ALS anyway. We use foods. The foods are going to be determined by the fat content in the membrane. There will be fatty foods to be avoided and foods that have fatty acids that will be recommended. Diet plays probably the most important part in the treatment and reversal of any of these diseases, particularly in this case.

While that's going on, we encourage the use of essential oils like lavender or lemon. There are other great oils such as frankincense. There's a mixture called Thieves made by a company called Young Living. Those were the essential oils we used in that particular case.

The microcurrents that were selected took into account the nerves themselves because we can focus on the anatomical parts of the body: the brain, the nerves, the musculature, and literally the cells themselves. Then we can program the equipment for the degenerative processes of something as serious as ALS. We can also program for the heavy metals that we assumed were part of it.

We never measured any metals in this patient. It seems odd that one of my first steps as a physician in the early days was to get heavy metal testing. We now assume that by the time you get a serious disease, it's due to heavy metals—at least in some part—so we don't have to test. We need to get on to detoxifying and removing them.

The clinical improvements that we watch as we detoxify will confirm that heavy metals played a role. When we set out to actually remove those metals, and the patient benefits, you're allowed to take the leap to say the detoxification helped bring about the improvement. As this patient improved, we felt that detoxification through multiple methods led to those improvements. What happened in that particular case can and usually does happen in other cases with regularity.

. . . .

Dr. Kondrot: For people who are reading this chapter, what recommendations do you have right now to improve their health?

Dr. Courtney: The best advice you can give to anyone is that if you are ill or have a set of disagreeable symptoms, you absolutely must have a plan that will help deal with toxicity issues. If your doctor is not conversant with this and recommends only the same medicine everybody else does, you need to break out of that mold and seek professional help from doctors who are comfortable with detoxing and removing heavy metal burden.

I often put it into a treatment triad with three prongs, and I call it the legs of a three-legged stool. One prong is to correct all deficiencies because they certainly have played a role in this person's disease process. The second prong is to remove all toxicities. It's absolutely certain, in any disease, that the patients have deficiencies and toxicities in combination, which have led them to whatever symptoms or disease they're presenting with. A third component that can't be ignored is the ability of the heart and blood vessels to bring an optimal amount of blood to any organ. The better you can improve profusion, the easier you will be able to correct a deficiency and remove toxicities. This is overlooked by many alternative doctors.

That treatment triad dominates my thinking processes every time I put a program together for any patient. That treatment triad is what I'd like people who read this chapter to leave with. If they put that program in play, they will improve; their symptoms will lessen; and their diseases will get better.

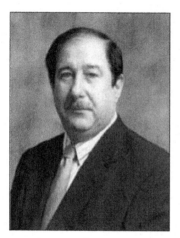

Dennis J. Courtney, MD

The Centers for Complementary Health

3075 Washington Road

McMurray, PA 15317

724-942-3002

www.djcmd.com

docdjc@gmail.com

RELEASE PHYSICAL AND MENTAL TOXINS THROUGH ENERGETIC TECHNIQUES

Interview with
Lee Cowden, MD, MD(H)

Chairman of the Scientific Advisory Board of the Academy of Comprehensive and Integrative Medicine and Academy Professor, Dr. Lee Cowden is a USA board-certified cardiologist and internist who is internationally known for his knowledge and skill in practicing and teaching integrative medicine. He has co-authored many books and articles on integrative medicine and has pioneered successful treatments for cancer, autism, Lyme disease, and many other illnesses.

1. Muscle testing taps into the autonomic nervous system in a simple way to learn things about the patient's body and the function of the body.

2. We have techniques to shake loose the cellular memory of trapped emotions and beliefs that cause a person to remain physically ill.

· ·

Dr. Kondrot: Please tell us about your medical training and how you became interested in chelation and detoxification.

Dr. Cowden: I went to medical school at the University of Texas, Houston, and after that, completed the internal medicine residency at St. Louis University Hospital Group in St. Louis. That was followed by critical care and cardiology fellowships at the St. Louis University Hospital and St. John's Mercy Medical Center in St. Louis. During my first few months in medical school, I became ill. I got advice from the chairmen of three different medical school departments. I followed their advice and got progressively worse.

My wife's grandmother came to visit us. She took me to the health food store and got me on some vitamins, minerals, and herbs, and then I got well fairly quickly. I determined, at that point, that I needed to learn what this woman knew about nutrition and take with a grain of salt the things I learned in medical training after that. I started reading very early in medical school about nutrition, detoxification, and things like that.

When I finished my formal training, I practiced conventional medicine for a year. I saw that this was not right because I knew about other things from my own reading and practice on family and friends. They were things that worked better than what I'd learned in conventional training, so I started using what I'd learned on my own more and more in practice and what I learned in my conventional training less and less.

In 1987, I moved to Dallas and set up a practice. It was a preventative cardiology practice, so I was seeing a lot of patients with chronic illness. There were patients who had all kinds of diagnostic labels, not just cardiovascular disease but also cancer, arthritis, and other serious conditions.

Very soon after that, I started doing muscle testing, a form of energetic testing. That helped me realize that an underlying cause for a lot of the problems I was seeing was the toxicity they had accumulated over the previous decades. That's when I started focusing more on detoxification, and I got better results with that.

Dr. Kondrot: Why has muscle testing become important in your process of evaluating a patient?

Dr. Cowden: Allopathic medicine primarily uses blood tests, other laboratory tests, and scanning procedures to determine what they're going to do about their patient's condition. The scanning procedures look primarily at the anatomy of the body. A couple of them only look at the function of the body. PET scanning, nuclear SPECT scanning, and functional MRI scanning look at function. The rest of them just look at anatomy, which is one of the last things that changes in a disease process. Then we use electrocardiograms and electroencephalograms, electromyograms, nerve conduction velocities, and other tests of the energy system of the body. The laboratory tests, blood tests, urine tests, and so on look a little further upstream at the disease process but not nearly as far upstream as the energetic evaluation of the body.

There are good ways to use the energy system of the body to find out what's going on besides the tests that are accepted in allopathic medicine. Those would be tests that look at the autonomic nervous system function of the body. There are a lot of tests that do that, like heart rate variability and so on. Muscle testing is a way to tap into the autonomic nervous system in a very inexpensive and simple way to learn things about the patient's body and the function of the body. You cannot get this same information from blood tests or scans because those allopathic tests are not sensitive enough to find the abnormalities you're looking for.

I started out with O-ring muscle testing, which means you oppose the thumb with an index, middle, ring, or pinky finger on the patient and see if you can pull the tightly held fingers apart. If you challenge the patient with something that is not agreeable to the body, whether it's a toxic substance, food allergen, or something else, their fingers fall apart. They develop a weakness in their fingers because the autonomic nervous system affects the muscle strength and the blood flow to the muscle. The change happens very quickly after the body is exposed to a toxic substance, food allergen, or anything else.

That response is also detectable by electrodermal screening, which is another tool I use in energetic testing. Electrodermal screening was developed by

Dr. Reinhard Voll in Germany in the 1950s. Many of his students have taken it to a new level with computerized technology and automated testing. With these techniques that primarily assess the autonomic nervous system, we can discover things about the patient that we have no way of finding out from a blood test, scans, or X-rays.

· ·

Dr. Kondrot: What do you feel is the most important information the public needs to know about detoxification?

Dr. Cowden: I have an analogy in the book I wrote recently on toxicity which is probably a good way for the people who are reading this book to understand what toxicity is. The analogy is that the toxic body is like a bathtub full of dirty water, and the dirty water is flowing over onto the bathroom floor. The bathtub represents the human body. The dirty water flowing onto the bathroom floor represents symptoms that have occurred because of the toxic buildup in that bathtub. The dirty water faucets are streaming dirty water into the bathtub. This dirty water includes nutrient-depleted foods, electromagnetic fields, radiation, pollution, toxic relationships, toxic emotions, tissue acidity, heavy metals, polluted air, antibiotics, pesticides, biotoxins, hypoxia, allergens, and other things. The clean water faucets at the top of the bathtub are mostly shut off, and hardly any clean water is flowing into the bathtub. They represent healthy foods and nutrients, purpose and will to live, sunshine, exercise, good relationships, peace, joy, love, a great attitude, restful sleep, pure water, and fresh air. The drains at the bottom of the tub are clogged up. They represent a toxic, constipated bowel, toxic liver and gallbladder, toxic kidneys, and a toxic, congested lymphatic system. The lymphatic system has tiny vessels that carry toxins away from the tissues. They're smaller than the veins and arteries that carry blood away from and to the tissues respectively.

In this analogy, in order for somebody to get well, they have to turn off the dirty water faucets and open up the clean water faucets that put more clean water into the bathtub. Then they have to open the drains at the bottom, so they can get well. When I teach other patients or practitioners how to do this, I say, "Focus on that analogy. Figure out what's putting the dirty water in, whether it's chemicals from the food or air, electromagnetic pollution from the environment, or toxic emotions. Try to start turning off some of those dirty water faucets." Once they've accomplished turning off the dirty water faucets, they can start opening up the clean water faucets, putting more good stuff in, and actively getting toxins out through the detox pathways of the bowel, liver, gallbladder, kidneys, lymphatics, and even the skin through a sauna. This analogy basically allows a patient to understand how to do things in a sequential sequence.

Another analogy is this: If you're in a rowboat in the middle of the ocean and you have a hole in the middle of your boat and your boat is taking on water, you don't just take a coffee cup and start dipping the water out. The first thing you do is plug the hole in the bottom of the boat. That stops the ongoing toxicity input into the body. Once you have the boat plugged, then you can detoxify and get the toxins out. Until you get the holes plugged, you can't have any hope of detoxifying.

A similar analogy would be a mouthful of mercury amalgams that are releasing microscopic mercury into your saliva and into the air you breathe every time you chew. How can you ever hope to get microscopic mercury out of your body until you get the mercury fillings out of your teeth?

. . . .

Dr. Kondrot: Because there are a myriad of toxins and environmental factors that are adversely affecting us, I think you have a very unique approach to detoxifying. Please go into some detail about your approach.

Dr. Cowden: When I first set up my practice in Dallas, I was using a lot of intravenous therapies because that's what I learned first as a way to remove heavy metals. I did intravenous EDTA chelation therapy. In my last office in Dallas, I had 20 recliners that people sat in while they got their intravenous EDTA chelation therapy and other nutritional therapies to detoxify their bodies. We ran two shifts a day, so sometimes we had 40 patients over the course of a day who got detoxification.

That was effective but very time-consuming for the patient because they were sitting there for about three hours. It was also very costly for the patients, and I felt that I needed to have a faster, less expensive way to do this that might also be even safer than that approach. What I figured out is energy medicine gets toxins out the fastest way, and you have to deal with the toxic emotions that cause the body to hold on to physical toxins if you want to have the greatest success. You have to use sufficient amounts of oral substances to bind toxins and remove them from the body through the bowel.

Let's say a heavy metal is mobilized out of the tissues. The heavy metals can be dumped into the bloodstream and carried by the bloodstream to the kidneys and then from the kidneys filtered into the urinary bladder and out the body. The same heavy metals can go from the bloodstream into the liver and be processed by the liver, dumped into the gallbladder and bile ducts, and then from there into the bowel. If you don't have anything in the bowel to bind the toxins, then they get reabsorbed through the bowel lining into the bloodstream and get recycled.

I figured out very early on that you need binding agents in the gut to be able to get toxins out, so I use a variety of things like chlorella and some of the clays and fibers to bind toxins in the bowel. I also use some of the metal binders that actually get into the bloodstream to bind things there.

Instead of using intravenous EDTA chelation therapy, I use the oral phospholipid-bound EDTA and other absorbable metal binders like DMSA and DMPS to bind the toxins in the tissues and carry them out of the body. Most importantly, I use an energy medicine approach to shake the toxins loose from the cells in the first place. I sometimes do the energy medicine part with homeopathic drops that the patient takes by mouth. Sometimes I also do that with a process called laser detox.

The laser detox is something I co-developed with two PhDs back in 2001. The laser detox is fairly rapid in its ability to remove toxins from the body. In my experience, it removes toxins about 20 times faster than the next closest competitive technique that I've identified so far. With the laser detox, you test the patient to find out what toxins are in their body. You make up a clear glass phial that contains those toxins in what's called a homeopathic homocord, which is a variety of different homeopathic dilutions all in one bottle. Then you shine a laser pointer through the clear glass phial onto the patient's body in a sweeping fashion. When you shine a laser pointer through a cylindrical clear glass phial, instead of the light coming out the other side as a point, it's actually a line. You can sweep that line over the body by moving it up and down, especially over the palms of the hands, the soles of the feet, and the ears. When you do that, the body starts releasing physical toxins from the cells into the space around the cells, the intracellular matrix. There, the lymphatic system and venous system can pick up those toxins and carry them back toward the central circulation.

From there, the toxins are sometimes bound by heavy metal binders that are taken by mouth—the EDTA, DMSA, DMPS, and so on. Sometimes the toxins are cleared out through the kidneys. Sometimes the toxins are cleared through the liver, gallbladder, and bowel. In order to prevent the reabsorption of toxins from the bowel, you need to have metal binders in the bowel, like chlorella, zeolite, and other clays and fibers. When you do this approach, because emotions have continued to hold on to those toxins, the toxins flood out fairly quickly.

I use other drainage remedies to support and strengthen the detox capability of the liver, gallbladder, kidneys, lymphatic system, and even clear toxins out of the ground matrix that's basically between the cells. In addition, it's very important to get the bowel working really well. Most people think if they're having a couple of bowel movements a week, they're okay. We really should have three bowel movements a day. Otherwise, we're considered to be constipated, and toxins will be recycled within our body.

. . . .

Dr. Kondrot: Your approach is more of an energetic approach using homeopathic dilutions which are essentially beyond any physical measurement to help remove the toxins.

Dr. Cowden: Right. The homeopathy works on the principle of like curing like. Dr. Samuel Hahnemann came up with that theory in about 1790. So far, it's borne out to be true that you can treat like with like. What that basically means is if you're poisoned with arsenic, the best treatment to get the arsenic out is homeopathically diluted arsenic. We use that principle very effectively in integrative medicine as part of the detoxification program, whether it's through homeopathic drops that the patient takes by mouth or rubs on the skin or whether it's by the laser detox.

. . . .

Dr. Kondrot: Please share a case that illustrates this approach, maybe someone who did not respond to conventional IV chelation.

Dr. Cowden: I'll tell you a case that illustrates the laser detox. I had a patient who had severe neuropathy, and he had gone to a variety of other doctors first. He went to an internist, a neurologist, and a neurosurgeon to figure out why he had this excruciating pins and needles sensation in his legs below his knees and why he couldn't feel his hand touching his leg in that area. He finally came to my office and said, "What do you think is causing this?" I said, "It's probably a toxin." When I did energy testing on him, we found that gasoline showed up as the toxin in his nervous system. I thought, "We'll see what happens." So we made up a homeopathic phial of gasoline with all the homeopathic dilutions necessary to get the gasoline toxin out of his body.

I put that phial in front of a laser pointer and handed it to an assistant. I said, "Go in that dark room and shine the laser pointer in this fashion over the patient's body. Come back out when you're finished." She went into the room and started shining the laser pointer on the patient's body and came back out gasping for breath. She said that the smell of gasoline was so strong that she couldn't stay in the room any longer. Less than a minute later, the patient came out and said, "You really need to get an exhaust fan in there." I stuck my head into the room, but I couldn't go in because it smelled so strongly of gasoline; all she had done was shine a light through a clear glass phial of a homeopathic homocord of gasoline onto his body, which caused the rapid release of gasoline from his cells into his bloodstream, which went to his lungs, and was released in his breath. Perhaps some was even coming out through his skin. We had to keep the room closed off for the rest of the day. Following that 30-second treatment, the symptoms of neuropathy were almost completely gone a month later. That illustrates how powerful energy medicine can be.

I've had patients who have gone through protracted intravenous chelation therapies to get heavy metals out of their body and then came to my practice to get help. The first day, we do laser energetic detox on them and give them the appropriate oral binders of the heavy metals, the lipophos EDTA, the DMSA, the zeolite, or chlorella. We collect a urine specimen afterward to see what came out. Usually we find that the heavy metals have just flooded out compared to the 24-hour urine collection they brought from the other practitioner who had been giving DMPS intravenously— sometimes for several weeks or months—before they came to my practice. It just illustrates how much more rapidly toxins can be removed from the body if you use energy medicine.

· ·

Dr. Kondrot: I know this is a very powerful technique, and you're actively involved in teaching other physicians how to use it. Please describe your role through the ACIM.

Dr. Cowden: The Academy of Comprehensive Integrative Medicine (ACIM) is an organization that includes health professionals as well as the general public. My desire is to reach as many health professionals as I can who are open-minded and interested in learning some of the things I've just talked about, so I can teach them what works well and let them use it for the betterment of their patients. The practitioners who become members of the academy can take online courses to learn a lot of this. They can start implementing some of the things they learn with their family, friends, and patients in a very short period of time. We also have webinars and live conferences. We teach practitioners through those means as well.

Recently, the academy has decided to start an online integrative medicine fellowship, so we'll have practitioners from all over the world coming together teaching certain materials. These will be in live conferences, but these live conferences will be filmed, edited, uploaded onto the academy website, and made into courses that can be streamed from the academy website by anybody in the world who wants to learn. Our goal is to start getting those courses translated into other languages like Spanish, Portuguese, French, German, and possibly others.

When practitioners start implementing these techniques in their practice, we want them to start collecting information about what they're accomplishing. Practitioners will ask their patients to complete a uniform questionnaire. It will be used in all the practices around the globe that use a particular methodology. When patients come back for follow up, they fill out a similar questionnaire, and we can compare the before and after subjective data on the patient, and collect certain objective findings through laboratory tests, scans, heart rate variability, and other testing that can show before and after changes. Very soon, we hope to show, on a worldwide scale, that what we're doing in integrative medicine works better than what's being used in allopathic medicine.

Dr. Kondrot: If patients who are reading this chapter are interested in finding a doctor who does the laser detoxification method, the best source would be the Academy of Comprehensive Integrative Medicine.

Dr. Cowden: Yes. On the website, we have a practitioner referral source. People who come to www.ACIMConnect.com can search for a practitioner closest to them geographically who has the knowledge to help them by using these techniques.

Inside the academy, we also have a mentoring system. If a person from the public contacts us with a very difficult problem, the academy tries to assist them to find the right help. Sometimes it will be through a person from another country who may not speak the same language as the patient. Through the academy website, we can actually set up an internet-based, three-way conversation between the patient, the practitioner who has been working with the patient, the expert practitioner, and a translator who will translate between the two practitioners. The teaching practitioner can hear the responses of the patient and may even ask some questions of the patient. The multi-direction teaching session goes on through the internet until the learning practitioner—the practitioner who is primarily responsible for the patient—has enough information to move ahead to try to help the patient.

They do that as many times as they need to until the patient is well. Sometimes we have to connect the practitioner to more than one mentor to help the patient. This process is the way things will be done in the future. The new medical paradigm will be based on reaching out internationally.

Dr. Kondrot: What can patients do right now to improve their health and detoxify?

Dr. Cowden: The first thing is to turn off the dirty water faucets at the top of their figurative bathtub. That means to clean up their diet. Don't eat junk foods. Eat live, whole foods, preferably sprouted and fermented foods predominantly. Make sure those foods are organic as much as possible and non-genetically modified. We know the genetic modification of foods causes all kinds of health challenges like leaky gut, cancers, autoimmune disease, and other things.

What we put into our body is critically important. If a person has limited financial resources, they would be wise to plant a garden in their backyard. If they live in a far northern climate and don't have many months of growing season, it would be wise to put an inexpensive greenhouse in their backyard to be able to grow year round. Then you would have good quality food that is organic and non-GMO and grown from native seeds. Your food will be harvested fresh, ripe, and ready to eat rather than picked green somewhere on the other side of the world and transported to you.

If you have limited financial resources, be sure the animal proteins you consume are all organic. It's more important to eat organic meats, dairy, eggs, and so on than it is to get organic vegetables and fruits because non-organic animal-derived proteins have anywhere from 5 to 20 times more pesticides and herbicides than organic vegetables. Animal protein can really contribute a huge toxic load through the diet.

Some people would be wise to reduce their animal source protein. So many people in the United States have kidney failure because they're getting way too much protein. The kidneys are getting toxic and overloaded from trying to process all that unnecessary protein, most of which goes into the gut and ferments, produces nitrosamines, and gets absorbed in the bloodstream. That makes the body toxic.

If you're going to improve your diet and digestion, you also need to do stress reduction techniques before meals so you have better hydrochloric acid production and better digestion capability in your stomach. Do things to get your bowels moving three times a day instead of twice a week. That includes taking magnesium and vitamin C. Toxins not dumped out with your bowel movements will be reabsorbed and poison your body.

Another thing that is important in getting people healthy is to reduce electromagnetic pollution. Electromagnetic pollution is disrupting the gut barrier. When you have microscopic holes in your gut barrier, the undigested proteins and other substances from your ingested foods can go through your gut wall back into the bloodstream and cause allergy and immune reactions which then distress your immune system.

Reduce exposure to electromagnetic fields. Simple things to do along those lines include turning off the circuit breakers that go to your bedroom. This will lower the electromagnetic field readings over your bed down to the lowest level you can get, which is what you have when the master breaker for the whole house is turned off. Turn off your breakers at night so you're not getting dirty electricity and 60 hertz electromagnetic pollution through the wall circuit.

Get rid of the cordless phone completely. Throw it away or give it to your worst enemy. Replace it with corded telephone lines. Make sure you keep your cell phone on airplane mode as much of the time as possible. Only take it off airplane mode briefly to check your voice and text messages. Turn it back on airplane mode after you've checked those messages. Return your phone calls from a landline whenever possible. If you can't return them from a landline, put your cell phone on speaker mode instead of holding it up to your ear. Put it just beyond the reach of your outstretched hand, and then shout at it.

These are simple things that almost anyone can do. Turn off your Wi-Fi at night. It's better to have only corded internet connections in your house, no wireless at all, as far as health goes.

If you live right down the street from a cell phone tower, get a German metalized cloth canopy to put over your bed or move because that is going to severely disrupt your gut barrier as well as your blood/brain barrier. When we have electromagnetic pollution in our environment, we develop leaks in the barrier between the bloodstream and the brain, which allow toxins to flood the brain. We wonder why we have a skyrocketing incidence of Alzheimer's and dementia in this country. It's my conclusion that it's primarily from the electromagnetic fields that people are exposed to.

The other thing I would have people do who are trying to get detoxified is figure out how to detoxify their emotions. I learned years ago that physical toxins are held onto in the body because of emotional toxins. The emotional toxins are not just the toxins you experience during your own lifetime but also the emotional toxins you pick up from your mom and dad while you're in mom's womb for nine months. They are still there.

The emotional toxins that have the greatest impact on physical health are those toxins we experience while we're in the womb for nine months. The second greatest impact from emotions is those emotions we experience in the first year of life. The third greatest impact from emotions is the emotions we experience in the second year of life. The fourth greatest is in the third year of life, and so on. By the time we're teenagers, the emotions we experience usually don't have a huge impact on our physical health but only upon our psyche and our emotional and mental health.

The way I usually get rid of the emotional toxins most rapidly in patients who have them contributing to physical toxicity is to use a combination of recall healing and EVOX. There are a variety of courses on www.ACIMConnect.com for recall healing. It's best done by somebody else, not by yourself. We're blinded to our own emotional baggage. We have to rely on somebody else to see that stuff for us and ask the right questions to shake loose the memory of emotional trauma and the decisions associated with it that cause our body to hold on to physical toxins.

EVOX is added to the recall healing because it makes the whole process faster and more efficient. EVOX is software from a company out of Salt Lake City, Utah—the ZYTO Corporation. It allows the patient to speak into a microphone, and the microphone records not the words but the vibrational frequencies embedded in the patient's voice. Each vibrational frequency corresponds to a specific emotion or belief related to the event or person that the patient is dwelling on or thinking about. After just 15 seconds of speaking into a microphone, you can see, displayed on a computer screen, all the emotions and beliefs you have related to a person or event. Seeing that on the screen causes the brain to start trying to process or release the emotions it was unaware of 15 seconds earlier.

The EVOX device goes a step beyond that and converts the voice frequencies of the patient into a homeopathic-like energy that it delivers back to the patient through an electrode the patient has their hand on while they're listening to pleasant music. This literally shakes loose the cellular memory of trapped emotions and beliefs that cause a person to remain physically ill.

What we usually see with a patient who goes through two or three sessions of recall healing and EVOX, which take about 45 minutes to an hour each, is that they have a huge dumping of emotional toxins which then usually causes a dumping of physical toxins as well.

That's why they need to have their bowel moving three times a day, have their lymphatic system cleaned out, and be on the appropriate oral toxin binders so they're binding up toxins in their gut before they even do the emotional release sessions.

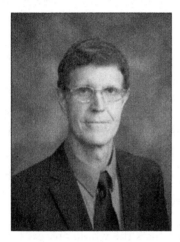

W. Lee Cowden, MD, MD(H)
Flower Mound, TX
www.ACIMConnect.com

DETOXIFICATION: MEDICINE FOR NOW AND THE FUTURE

Interview with
Martin Dayton, DO

Dr. Martin Dayton has been practicing chelation therapy since 1979. He has been licensed as an osteopathic physician in Florida since 1971. He has earned two doctorates in medicine, DO and MD. His undergraduate work was in agriculture and environmental science. He has held various university professorial positions and is a researcher, clinician, and teacher.

1. When a person is in harmony, the person is at ease; the opposite of ease is *dis-ease*.

2. A person with mercury toxicity may be tired or have brain fog. People have much greater clarity after undergoing chelation therapy.

3. I think chelation therapy will become standard care in the future because the studies and statistics are quite favorable.

Dr. Kondrot: Please tell us a little bit about your medical training and how you became interested in chelation and detoxification.

Dr. Dayton: My medical training started in undergraduate school. I attended Rutgers College of Agriculture and Environmental Science and studied what makes living systems healthy and what makes them perform and heal better. Then I went into culture shock. I went to medical school where there was a concentration on pharmaceutical medicine.

In my center now, we do three things to try to improve harmony and balance in a person. One is to reduce or eliminate those factors that prevent optimal function and repair. Such factors can be maladaptive thoughts as well as toxic metals. We also try to improve the mineral integrity and the general balance of the person spiritually, physically, and emotionally. Second, we try to determine what is deficient. There could be deficiency in spontaneity or in various nutrients.

The third area I look at is the integration of all these different aspects of the person, so the person is in synchronous harmony. When a person is in harmony, the person is at ease. The opposite of ease is *dis-ease*, so the idea is to get rid of what doesn't belong, keep what does, and have everything integrate and move harmoniously. That is what is emphasized in addressing various conditions, at least from the standpoint of underlying causes.

Chelation is one way of reducing and eliminating toxicity, which prevents optimal function and repair. In chelation for metals, the idea is to reduce the toxic metallic influence and, in doing so, allow the body to improve and use its own innate healing abilities. Chelation therapy also involves essential metals. For example, if magnesium bound to EDTA is introduced into the body, EDTA exchanges the magnesium, which is an essential mineral, for a toxic metal such as lead. It carries the toxic metal out of the body via urine or stool. In chelation therapy, we are ridding the body of toxins, which prevent optimal function and repair. We also may add substances that are helpful for this same purpose.

Dr. Kondrot: Please give an example of your approach to treating a patient using those three areas to illustrate your method.

Dr. Dayton: Evaluation of the patient is subject to many factors. Those factors involve the desires and beliefs of the patients, the means of the patients, and the options available to the patient. Some might be limited by supply. Others might be limited by cost. We try to tailor the approach to what best fits a patient's needs.

If we're looking for nutritional deficiencies, there are various tests available to determine the presence and spectrum of fatty acids, minerals, vitamins, and amino acids. We take various samples from the body, including urine, hair, blood, and saliva. We look at the body's components and use this information to try to improve general balance to overcome deficiencies. We also look to see what toxic stuff may be in the body. For example, we check for toxic metals such as cadmium, lead, and mercury. Some metals are conditionally toxic, such as calcium, iron, and copper. These metals are essential, but when they are present in excess, they can become toxic. Some metals, such as mercury, are always toxic.

We look for the presence of other types of toxins that may be in the body, like microtoxins that come from mold. The world is very toxic. We have organic toxins, not just metallic toxins, to deal with.

Once we evaluate for toxicity in the body, we look to see what else may be interfering with the person's well-being. Some of it is psychological. There is a physician named Eric Berne who was quite a famous psychiatrist in his day. He felt that once we are able to meet our basic needs such as breathing, eating food, drinking water, and such, three things are needed to be happy, or at least to enjoy life. One had to do with spontaneity. Another had to do with appreciation of one's surroundings or awareness. The third had to do with intimacy. He suggested that if we had those three, we'd enjoy life. Many people with disease, unfortunately, are not enjoying life. If they improve the balance of the three areas of awareness, spontaneity, and intimacy, they may find their quality of life considerably improved.

· ·

Dr. Kondrot: During the course of your evaluation and treatment, do you educate people on those three areas to help them achieve health and happiness?

Dr. Dayton: Yes. We pay attention to those areas and various things that can disturb the appreciation of life. For example, resentment, regret, and self-righteousness may interfere with the ability to enjoy life, so we look for disturbances in the psyche and try to overcome those as well as look at deficiencies. We find that chelation therapy is not the only way to address factors which prevent optimal function and repair.

· ·

Dr. Kondrot: I think your approach is unique in that you're not only look-ing at the physical causes of toxicity in the body but also at aspects that might affect the psychological well-being. Can you give an example of a patient you treated using this comprehensive approach?

Dr. Dayton: We have many patients, and each and every one is an individual. For example, mercury toxicity affects many aspects of a person. A person with mer-cury toxicity might manifest rashes, burning pain in the body, an up-and-down personality, or emotional instability. Various infections or other immune issues may manifest. A person with mercury toxicity may present as tired or having brain fog. We not only use chelation to remove the mercury, but on the way to getting better, there are various issues people have to address. Very often, I discuss the in-teraction of mercury with the personality. I had one patient who was detoxed for mercury. During detox, he actually hit somebody with a garbage bag and had no idea why. It was explained to him that it was probably part of his mercury detox. As he continued to detox, his personality became more normal and he did very well.

· ·

Dr. Kondrot: What do you feel is the essential information that the public should be aware of about chelation and detox?

Dr. Dayton: Chelation is only one part of a puzzle, but it's an important part. For example, chelation could play a part in six of the seven leading causes of death. Those are heart disease, cancer, lower respiratory diseases, stroke, Alzheimer's, and diabetes. Those are the causes one through seven minus one. The fifth leading cause has to do with accidental injuries. Of the six causes I mentioned, chelation has been documented to favorably affect each one. There are no studies that have looked at accidental injuries relative to chelation. If you can significantly reduce the need for bypass surgeries, stenting, and some of the other potentially harmful therapies by using chelation therapy, I think it would contribute to reducing the risk of medical injuries.

There are studies showing that chelation therapy dramatically reduces the chances of having heart attacks and strokes in diabetics. It reduces the severity of diabetes mellitus. There was one study done over the course of 18 years where one group received chelation therapy and the other did not. The two groups were matched for similar characteristics. Eighteen years later, the research showed a tenfold decrease in cancer death rate among the patients who had chelation therapy versus those who did not. The idea is if you reduce toxic material early, you can theoretically prevent the expression of chronic degenerative diseases, including heart disease and cancer.

Chelation can affect various aspects of a person's life. We find that dementia can improve. People have much greater clarity after undergoing chelation therapy. Performance may improve. For patients who have severe peripheral vascular disease, it's been shown to dramatically reduce the need for amputation.

Dr. Kondrot: Are there certain chelating methods you prefer, depending on the heavy metal or toxin that's involved?

Dr. Dayton: For cardiovascular diseases and autoimmune diseases, I generally prefer EDTA plus magnesium, unless, through testing, we find that there's a spectrum of toxic metals that might be better addressed using a different chelating agent. What I like about the use of EDTA plus magnesium is that it reduces excess calcium, which can cause degenerative changes. Harmfully distributed calcium can interact negatively with toxic metals. Magnesium EDTA also removes toxic lead, cadmium, and a few others.

If the person has mercury toxicity, although EDTA does bind well with mercury, it does not remove it very well because the EDTA competes with the body's own tissues, which may have a greater affinity for holding on to mercury. For mercury toxicity, we use other substances such as DMPS or DMSA.

We try to fit the chelating agent and the regimen we use to each person's needs. Some patients do not want to undergo intravenous therapy while others are willing to do so. Depending upon test results and what best meets the patient's desires, we individualize our programs.

We try to put together regimens that make sense using both natural chelators such as those found in food as well as pharmaceutical ones. Nutritional supplements are helpful in addressing toxicity. For a person with mercury toxicity, I recommend sulfur-containing food such as eggs, onions, garlic, and cilantro. The nutrient lipoic acid is also helpful in reducing mercury. Other substances include zeolite and folic acid. We may use a number of them, sometimes concomitantly. To prevent reabsorption of mercury from the intestinal tract, we may use supplemental seaweed and modified citrus pectin.

· ·

Dr. Kondrot: Why do you think that there is so much resistance to chelation and detoxification?

Dr. Dayton: We're in a society where patients want immediate symptomatic results and where emphasis is placed more on the treatment of symptoms rather than the underlying causes. The pharmaceutical industry promotes the use of patented drugs. It's very profitable. Patents on chelating pharmaceuticals have usually expired, therefore reducing profits. Chelation therapy also diminishes profits from bypass surgery, arterial stenting, and other invasive procedures promoted by the lucrative cardiovascular industry.

The medical schools are under the influence of pharmaceutical companies. Medical literature is also under the influence of pharmaceutical companies. There is a financial incentive to ignore detoxification processes such as chelation in medical schools and in published medical literature.

The use of detoxification certainly would address many issues. I mentioned mercury toxicity where you might have a person manifesting rashes, burning pains in the extremities, brain fog, fatigue, personality issues, or concurrent infections. If the person were treated with contemporary conventional medicine, different pharmaceutical medicines would be used for each of those problems. The patient would end up with many pharmaceutical medicines, some used to overcome the effects of others. If we could detoxify mercury, all these issues would disappear. However, the orientation in medicine is not to look for underlying toxicity unless it is overwhelmingly acute.

Doctors are not taught in medical school to address underlying toxicity in the chronic conditions which exhibit a multitude of manifestations. They are taught to look at specific resulting diseases and then prescribe a symptomatic remedy. If we look for underlying toxicity as a way of addressing health and disease, we can eliminate many of the diseases or at least prevent many of them from occurring prematurely.

It takes a long time for medicine to change, and that is one good reason why we are still stuck in treating end results, signs, and symptoms rather than the disease process that underlies them. Through history, we have had examples of this. Dr. Ignaz Semmelweis, an Austrian gynecologist and obstetrician, presented a treatise about antiseptic procedures and the delivery of babies in 1861. He collected data for about ten years. As a reward for giving to the world the fruits of his labors and his genius, he was ostracized by the medical community, lost his job, and ultimately died after a mental breakdown in 1865. He was talking about cleansing, which is what chelation does. Two years later, another physician, Dr. Joseph Lister, also started to use cleansing techniques, but in surgery, and was also attacked by his colleagues. His saving grace was that a fellow named Louis Pasteur came on the scene and made the concept of germs popular. Then the medical profession was able to accept Dr. Lister's work.

Today, detoxification advocates still are being attacked. Recently, studies supported by a $30 million NIH grant were published through Mt. Sinai Hospital in Miami Beach. Dr. Gervasio Lamas, a renowned researcher at Mt. Sinai, found chelation statistically to be very helpful in reducing the incidence of heart attacks and death due to heart attack in the relatively large population he studied. We have had much less criticism about chelation therapy since these studies came out.

. . . .

Dr. Kondrot: We need to educate the public, and I think you're to be congratulated on the book you wrote, *The Case for Intravenous Chelation Therapy,* **which is a very useful handbook for helping patients understand chelation. What else do you feel physicians need to do to bring this important message to patients?**

Dr. Dayton: As an aside, that book was used to acquire the National Institute of Health grants to do the studies coordinated via Mount Sinai. The studies were done not only at Mount Sinai but also at many sites, including at some of the more prestigious institutions in the United States.

Doctors need to educate their patients, but they also need to educate themselves. There's still a lot of stigma about chelation therapy. It's been maligned for many years, and it takes a while for the medical profession to overcome its inertia. While we do have studies done by credible institutions now, it's a matter of publishing more studies. Dr. Lamas is about to embark on more studies. He's been able to put studies together that are more acceptable to most physicians. As chelation becomes more accepted and shown to be economically feasible, especially compared to standard care alone, insurance will begin to pay for it. Presently, insurance companies covering chelation for conditions like cardiovascular disease and diabetes are relatively few. Once chelation therapy is approved by insurance, it will grow by leaps and bounds. Physicians previously opposed will offer it for better patient outcomes and financial profit.

Underlying disease, are various factors that prevent optimal function and repair. If we can address these issues through nutrition and chelation, we can help overcome disease that is now occurring and prevent the premature expression of other conditions. I think chelation therapy will become standard care in the future because the studies and statistics based on these studies are quite favorable.

In regard to doing chelation, nearly everyone on Earth may potentially benefit from detoxification because the earth is so polluted. If we continually cleanse ourselves of those factors that prevent our ability to function optimally and replenish factors that are necessary, we will function better. One of our innate capacities is to self-heal. Chelation therapy is not only remedial. I think it's also anti-aging. Chelation therapy, in my mind, is an excellent strategy for increasing a healthy life span.

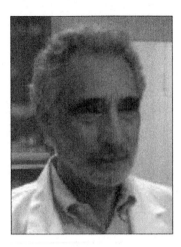

Martin Dayton, DO
Dayton Dandes Medical Center
18600 Collins Avenue
Sunny Isles Beach, FL 33160
305-931-8484
contact@daytondandesmedical.com
www.daytondandesmedical.com

CHELATION AND OTHER DETOX METHODS CAN SAVE YOUR LIFE

Interview with
Pieter DeWet, MD, MD(H), FAAFP, ABIHM

Dr. Pieter J. DeWet has been practicing wellness medicine since 1997 and is the owner and medical director of Quantum Healing Institute in Tyler, TX. Dr. DeWet graduated medical school in 1985. He has been a diplomat of the American Board of Holistic and Integrative Medicine since the year 2000. In 2007, he received his Arizona homeopathic and integrative medicine license.

Dr. DeWet completed his residency in family medicine at the University of Texas Health Center at Tyler in 1991 where he was intimately involved in the development of numerous chronic disease management programs. He was also the founder and director of the Center for Nutrition and Preventive Medicine there from 1995 to 1997.

Dr. DeWet has spent his entire career searching for the most effective, least harmful, and the most cost-effective methods to treat patients with complex health challenges. He currently treats patients from all around the country and worldwide for diseases and health conditions ranging from the most simple to some of the most complex. Dr. DeWet approaches all patients holistically, which means he focuses on body, mind, and soul and routinely addresses and assists in the treatment of a patient's physical, emotional, social, mental, environmental, and spiritual issues as they relate to their overall health. He is determined to find and treat the root causes of illness in each patient. For this reason Dr. DeWet is credited for getting very good results with the majority of his patients, especially those who commit to healing all aspects of their health challenges.

1. **All illnesses are triggered by unresolved conflicts that become biological.**

2. **Each part of the brain and each organ or tissue is impacted by specific conflicts and emotion.**

3. **There's no such thing as an incurable illness. Even Ebola or rabies has cure rates of at least 50 percent.**

· ·

Dr. Kondrot: Please tell us a little bit about your medical training and how you became interested in chelation and detoxification.

Dr. DeWet: I attended medical school in South Africa and got my MD degree in 1985. I spent a year doing a rotating internship in South Africa, and I came to the United States in 1987. My goal was to learn more about holistic and integrative medicine. Even while attending medical school, I had a strong desire to learn more about holistic medicine and what really caused disease. I read books and completed courses outside of my medical school training. I understood the limitations of conventional medicine's almost exclusive focus on symptom management and disease management, and I had a burning desire to learn as much as I could about natural and holistic approaches to healing right from the start.

After I got to the United States, I connected with a great mentor, Dr. David Steenblock, and spent 18 months working with him and learning as much as I could about integrative medicine. In order to pursue further training, I had to get my license in the United States, which meant three years of post-graduate training, which I did in family practice. In 1991, coming out of residency, I was invited to join the faculty at the University of Texas Health Center in Tyler—now called the University of Texas Health North East. I spent seven years in academic medicine teaching other physicians and training medical students. At the university, I was able to pursue my passion for integrative medicine by taking the lead in starting a new department called the Center for Nutrition and Preventative Medicine. When I left there, I entered private practice in order to pursue my dream to practice a more unrestricted form of integrative medicine and to be able to make a more profound difference. My practice in Tyler, Texas, has gone through a series of meta-morphoses over the past 17 years as I have learned more and adjusted my approach to healing to become increasingly holistic. The facility is now called Quantum Healing Institute (QHI Wellness).

Since I left medical school, I've attended dozens of medical conferences on in-tegrative and natural medicine. I've learned from some of the world's top minds in the integrative medical field. I have studied homeopathy, homotoxicology, IV and oral chelation therapy, herbal medicine, orthomolecular medicine, bio-oxidative therapies, acupuncture, segment therapy, prolozone therapy, Recall Healing, hyp-nosis, Reiki, and many other modalities. I am board certified in family medicine and a diplomat of the American Board of Integrative and Holistic Medicine.

In the year 2000, I received my certification in chelation therapy through the American College for Advancement in Medicine (ACAM). Then over the years, I've learned a lot more about detoxification and chelation through various courses in integrative medicine.

. . . .

Dr. Kondrot: Was there a defining moment early in your medical training that made you realize that traditional Western medicine was not the best way to help patients?

Dr. DeWet: I was raised by parents who kept us away from conventional medicine. Instead they kept us healthy and used homeopathic, chiropractic, and natural medicine when we did get sick. My father was a chiropractor and an ex-traordinary healer who practiced in South Africa at a time when his profession was under siege by the conventional medical community, just like it was here in the United States in the '70s. He is the one who advised me not to go into chiropractic because of the challenging politics surrounding his profession at the time. Instead he encouraged me to get my medical degree which he thought would give me the freedom to practice "the best medicine I could" with a license that would allow me to add other integrative modalities.

My intention right from the start when I entered medical school was to become a holistic physician eventually. I knew I had to toe the line going through medical school and post graduate training, while still holding on to my intention and desire to learn about and contemplate the real causes of disease and how best to treat them.

· ·

Dr. Kondrot: What do you feel is really the important information that the public should know about chelation and detox?

Dr. DeWet: We live in a very toxic world. We are exposed to literally thousands of different toxins on an ongoing basis. Even though, in many ways, we have cleaner air and water than we had decades ago, there is a constant and growing onslaught of manmade toxins in everything from our food supply to our environment. Even in the medical and dental professions, we see more toxicities being introduced in the form of disease-causing drugs and toxic materials used in and on the body. These toxins include everything from heavy metals to pesticides, herbicides, solvents, toxic fumes, food additives, GMO foods, etc.

These toxins contribute to ill health in many different ways, and, in order to restore health and prevent disease, it is critical to reduce exposure to these toxins. Chelation therapy, for example, is one very helpful tool used for the removal of heavy metal toxins from the body. Heavy metal toxicity is becoming a bigger and bigger problem, contributing to damage of organ systems, such as the cardiovascular system, brain, nervous system, the kidneys, the immune system, bone marrow, and many others.

Each heavy metal has its own range of toxic effects and affects certain organ systems more than others. For example, aluminum toxicity has been implicated in neurological conditions, such as Alzheimer's and in certain kidney diseases. Aluminum is found in consumer products, including antiperspirants, cosmetics, and astringents, and as a food additive in baking powder. Just about everywhere you turn, there's aluminum in something. It is even used in drugs, such as antacids, buffered aspirin, and as a coating to make the medications look attractive. Aluminum compounds are used in many diverse and important industrial applications, such as alums (aluminum sulfate) used in water-treatment and alumina in abrasives and furnace linings.

Most people have mercury in their bodies. It is poisonous even in small amounts and commonly affects everything from the nervous system, including the brain, to the immune system and cardiovascular system. We know there's a great deal of exposure to this heavy metal as a result of the use of amalgams by the dental community that continues virtually unabated to this day. There's mercury in air pollution, especially from coal-burning power stations in China that is blown to the United States by the prevailing winds. There's mercury being emitted through smokestacks where they incinerate bodies, and our oceans and fresh water lakes are full of mercury as a result of this pollution. As a result, a lot of the fish we eat today is contaminated with mercury. Even vaccines often still contain mercury as a preservative, and eye drops used to clean contact lenses often contain it as well.

Lead toxicity contributes to many different diseases including neurological disorders and cardiovascular diseases, such as atherosclerosis and congestive heart failure. Lead is now found in every human being on the planet and is very difficult to remove from the body without some form of chelation. Sources of lead toxicity include paint containing lead that was used in older homes, petroleum products— even though leaded gasoline has been banned, etc. Other common heavy metal toxins that can have detrimental effects on our health include cadmium, arsenic, palladium, and radioactive heavy metals like uranium, strontium, plutonium, and radium. Many of the radioactive metals we are exposed to originate from nuclear disaster sites, such as Fukushima in Japan and Chernobyl in the Ukraine.

Our children are experiencing even greater levels of heavy metal toxicity. In our pediatric population, we often see more metals and other toxins as a result of exposure in the womb from the mother's body and in breast milk. Children are also exposed to these toxins from our contaminated food supply and our toxic environment. Add to that vaccines that contain mercury (the flu vaccine), aluminum, and other toxins, and you quickly can see how vulnerable our children can be. Even though mercury has been removed from many childhood vaccines, the flu vaccine still contains it.

We see a steadily worsening epidemic of chronic illnesses including numerous degenerative conditions, such as Alzheimer's, Parkinson's disease, and dementia. I believe metal toxicity and other toxins play a large role as contributing factors to those illnesses. Chelation therapy and other detoxification strategies are all helpful and often critical in reestablishing good health and preventing disease in those fortunate enough to be healthy.

. . . .

Dr. Kondrot: It's kind of scary when you go through that list of all those toxic metals we're being exposed to. What is your experience about how this affects us?

Dr. DeWet: My experience is that every one of the patients I see in my practice, regardless of what conditions they come in with, is toxic. I test all of them for toxicity as a routine part of my workup, and I routinely employ detoxification strategies and educate patients on how to reduce their exposure to environmental and waterborne and foodborne toxins. Failure to do so, in my experience, leads to poor results.

We know that certain metals, such as mercury, lead, cadmium, palladium, and radioactive heavy metals, such as plutonium, thorium, strontium 89, and uranium 235 are toxic to humans and animals even in small amounts and have been implicated in a great number of health challenges. Other metals, such as aluminum, gadolinium, nickel, tin, and titanium are also toxic but in larger amounts. Mercury, for example, is a neurotoxin and also causes damage to the immune system. The bottom line is there is no such thing as a safe mercury level. The same applies to lead and the radioactive metals.

Another important fact to consider is that certain heavy metals are not only poisonous by themselves, but when combined are even worse. For example, lead, mercury, and cadmium in the same person cause synergistic damage to his or her body. In experiments performed on rats, the amount of mercury that would kill one out of a hundred rats (LD1), when combined with the amount of lead and cadmium that would kill one out of a hundred rats, kills all of them (LD100) when combined together at those same levels.

Lead affects the cardiovascular system contributing to atherosclerosis, coronary artery disease, and congestive heart failure as well as the digestive tract, nervous system, fertility, etc. In fact, the chelating agent EDTA (ethylene diamine tetra-acetic acid) that was originally developed to assist in the detox of lead after lead poisoning was also found to be helpful in the treatment of cardiovascular diseases in those with lead poisoning. It surprisingly worked even in those without significant lead poisoning.

Heavy metals are difficult to clear out of the body because most of them have relatively long half-lives. Lead, for example, accumulates in the bones, and it can take seven-plus years just to get that lead out of the bones, even if you chelate somebody with EDTA regularly for that entire period of time. The half-life of lead without chelation is 70 years and that of mercury in the central nervous system is 15 to 30 years. These are difficult poisons to clear from the body. Combined with all the other poisons, pesticides, herbicides, and chemicals that get into our bodies, they all play a role in development of virtually every chronic disease we see, if not all of them.

· ·

Dr. Kondrot: Do you have a unique approach in terms of evaluating and treating patients whom you suspect may have heavy metal poisoning?

Dr. DeWet: First and foremost at QHI Wellness, we do a thorough evaluation to determine the patient's specific health challenges and to establish possible contributing factors. This includes a comprehensive history and physical to establish clinically supported diagnoses followed by appropriate conventional testing, including blood work. The history we perform includes a thorough evaluation of stress factors and underlying emotional conflicts behind disease (Recall Healing). Blood work, for example, on those suspected of cardiovascular disease or who are thought to be at risk for this often includes evaluation of advanced risk factors above and beyond the analysis of lipids; it may encompass evaluation for nutrient deficiencies, evaluation of key hormones, and evaluation for metal toxicities, including iron and copper.

When appropriate, especially in those who have or may have cardiovascular conditions, further tests may include heart rate variability analysis, EKG, echocardiograms, carotid sonograms, cardiac stress tests, etc. Most patients whom we see also undergo bio-energetic testing to highlight other potential contributors to ill health or risk factors that may cause problems. If heavy metal toxicity is suspected either clinically and/or based on bioenergetic testing, further testing for metals may follow, including blood tests, hair analysis, or a chelation challenge test with EDTA, DMSA, and/or other chelators followed by stool and urine analysis for metals. If we use IV chelators for this purpose, we may do testing after three IV chelations. This is done in order to clear the kidneys of heavy metals in order to obtain a more accurate test.

If heavy metal toxicity is proven to be a problem and if the diagnosis supports it, treatment commences. We take a multipronged approach in getting these toxins out of the body. Most importantly, the patient's diet is evaluated and dramatically reformed, if necessary. For example, we discourage the intake of refined carbohydrates, starchy vegetables, sugars as well as all genetically modified (GMO) foods. We encourage the elimination of all processed foods and those containing artificial sweeteners, coloring and flavoring agents, and preservatives. We recommend organic, pesticide and fungicide free foods, including vegetables, fruits, nuts, seeds, beans, and free range organic meats and eggs.

As far as getting heavy metals out of the body, we use various chelators and chelation methods, including IV and oral, depending on the patient, the diagnosis, and the severity of illness. Everything from traditional EDTA chelation therapy to other chelators, such as dimercaptosuccinic acid (DMSA) and 2,3-dimercapto-1-propanesulfonic sodium (DMPS), and a number of other natural chelators, such as chlorophyll-containing foods or superfoods such as chlorella and spirulina to support the detox pathways inside the body and inside the cells.

We use glutathione and numerous other nutrients, such as R-lipoic acids, N-acetylcysteine (NAC), CoQ10, the full complement of tocotrienols, tocopherols, and vitamin C to facilitate the removal of metals. We also use IV vitamin C as a weak chelator in those who are very ill and whom we suspect may have difficulty tolerating more aggressive IV chelation therapy at first. Other chelators include zeolite, seaweed extracts, cilantro, and certain homeopathics to support heavy metal detox. Aggressive mineral and trace mineral replacement and replenishment are also instituted in those getting chelation of any kind. Magnesium is one of those and is given intravenously along with IV chelators and also orally or transdermally. Most of those dealing with chronic illnesses or under a lot of stress have significant magnesium deficiencies. Zinc, manganese, chromium, molybdenum, copper, and selenium are also often given intravenously or orally along with other nutrients.

Laser energetic detoxification (LED) and far infrared pulsar therapy developed by Lee Cowden, MD, with the support of others, are also employed in many patients. This combines light energy or laser energy with homeopathic frequencies of the toxins that we are intent on clearing from the body. This involves the projection of a green or red laser beam through a vial filled with liquid containing the imprinted homeopathic frequencies of these toxins which is then administered to the surface of the body (acupuncture points and meridians) via this laser beam.

Other general strategies are used to support healing including probiotics and in those with leaky gut syndrome (increased gut permeability disorder); strategies are employed to repair the gut lining, including such remedies as Aloe vera, L-glutamine, and licorice root extract. Many patients also need support for proper digestion with digestive enzymes, bile, and hydrochloric acid replenishment with meals, all of which are critical in order to digest the food that we eat properly, making sure the body absorbs nutrients and can successfully remove toxins from the body.

Bio-oxidative therapies also play a critical role in speeding detox and repair in many. We use oxygen enrichment strategies such as nighttime oxygen supplementation in those with nocturnal hypoxia. Ozone, IV hydrogen peroxide, hyperbaric oxygen therapy (HBOT), and exercise with oxygen therapy (EWOT) are also used for their supportive effects on energy production in the body and also to help clear out toxins by supporting key detox pathways. Ozone is administered via IV infusion mixed with blood or via direct IV push, rectally, transdermally, intradermally, or directly in the bladder or vagina, for example. We also use a device called the HOCATT (hyperthemic ozone and carbonic acid transdermal therapy) that combines far infrared therapy with hyperthermia, ozone, EWOT, light therapy, carbonic acid, aromatherapy, and electrotherapy as part of our detox protocol. Ion foot cleanse technologies also facilitate detox.

In addition, I encourage my patients to do home-based detox protocols. Those include far infrared saunas, the supplements listed earlier, and lymph drainage enhancement strategies. Many of my patients have portable saunas or freestanding far infrared saunas at home. All patients are also instructed on how to optimize lymph drainage through dry skin brushing, rebounding, certain breathing techniques, and exercise.

We also use strategies that focus on the deeper roots of illness. One of the concepts I convey to patients, usually at their first visit, is to help them understand that disease often manifests on the physical level, but the root cause is often much deeper. I teach my patients that there are five levels of healing, drawn from the teachings of Dr. Dietrich Klinghardt. They include the physical body, energy body, mental body, intuitive body, and spirit body. Most of medicine focuses exclusively on the physical body and ignores the other four. I will briefly touch on these with excerpts from my book, *Heal Thyself: Transform Your Life, Transform Your Health*.

Energy Body: This level is the level linked to physics and physiology. The physical body is surrounded and penetrated by an energy field, which consists of electromagnetic, gravitational, weak nuclear and strong nuclear forces as well as light emissions. This level is affected by a variety of modern technologies, which are contributing tremendously to the ill health of individuals and to society as a whole. Devices, such as smart meters, cordless phones, Wi-Fi systems, electrical devices and wiring in our homes, microwave ovens, cell phones, and cell phone towers have some of the most devastating effects. Irradiation due to nuclear contamination, X-ray radiation from diagnostic devices, light pollution, and scars on the body affecting meridian energy flow also come into play on this level.

Mental Body: This level is linked to our belief systems, thoughts, feelings, and perceptions, which, in turn, organize our emotions and other aspects of the energy body. This body is both individualized and, at the same time, linked to and influenced by mass consciousness or consensus reality. Unresolved psychological conflicts (feelings buried alive) stemming from the traumatic experiences of our lives affect us at this level and form the root of most illnesses, especially when you add to that the conflicts we inherit through our genealogy and the conflicts we take on that relate to mass consciousness (level 4). Erroneous belief systems also form a key component that leads to dysfunction at this level.

I use a modality in my practice called Recall Healing, which is aimed at discovering and clearing the roots of illness at the mental body and intuitive body levels. The key concept behind Recall Healing is that virtually all illnesses are triggered by unresolved conflicts that become biological. A conflict initially occurs at a psychological level. As long as the conflict remains psychological, we remain healthy on a physical level; we become ill when the conflict becomes biological. Therefore, a biological conflict is an unresolved psychological conflict expressed in the body. When a conflict reaches a certain intensity where it threatens to overwhelm waking consciousness and the brain can no longer manage the body properly because of the amount of energy it is expending due to the psychological stress, the conflict is pulled down into the body—into the biology—and is transposed by the brain into the area that corresponds to the exact tonality of the conflict. In other words, each part of the brain and each organ or tissue is impacted by specific conflicts and emotion. Every physical illness is preceded by a triggering conflict. These can link up in different ways.

In Recall Healing, we look at no fewer than three layers of downloads that can lead to illness. The first layer includes those traumatizing events that take place starting about the first year of life through the present that lead to programming conflicts, further aggravated by subsequent triggering conflicts.

The second layer of downloads and the second major source of biological conflict, your project purpose, is set by one year of age and comes directly from your biological parents. Every person has a purpose that corresponds to the project that was made for it by its creator, which in a human being would be the biological parents. This programming is linked to the period starting nine months before conception through our first year of life. This is another survival tool and is essential for the parents to be able to function at a level in this world where they have the greatest chance of being able to support their offspring and continue to procreate. The unresolved psychological conflicts of the parents become the biological conflicts of the child.

The third layer of downloads we receive when we come into this world are downloads related to our genealogy and the transfer of family memories from one generation to another going back as far as four generations. This phenomenon is also called "biological cascades."

Key concepts in Recall Healing as discovered by Dr. Ryke Hamer:

1. The brain is the central control station, and illness is a program that the brain can switch on under circumstances of extreme stress or a very significant conflict.

2. The brain can switch off this same illness-creating program as soon as the conflict that triggered the illness has been resolved or is eliminated.

3. There is a consistent and profound link between the symbolism of illnesses, the part of the body that is affected, and the corresponding parts of the brain.

4. Every so-called disease has to be understood as a "meaningful, special biological program of nature" created to solve an unexpected, biological conflict. Disease, therefore, is not a fault, but an adaptation.

Intuitive Body: This level relates to the collective unconscious, also called mass consciousness. Not only do we carry our own individual unresolved conflicts, but we also carry the conflicts of our genealogy, our cultures, ethnicity, races, our communities, religions, and even of humanity as a whole. The most important conflicts to track down relate to our genealogy going back four generations including us. Any conflicts that led to a loss of love, respect, or intimacy need to be tracked down, if possible. Also critical is to acknowledge and bring to light family secrets and to heal the wounds left by devastating losses of loved ones in past generations.

Spirit Body: This is the level of religion and spirituality and the level of self-healing. One must overcome spiritual destitution in order to create an overarching framework for healing. This level of healing requires us to go within in order to connect with our creator and our divine essence, the ultimate source of healing. This is the level of unconditional love, ecstasy, unbridled joy of being, inner peace despite our health situations or life circumstance, and the feeling of oneness with all and our creator, of enlightenment, and pure consciousness. If this is achieved, then healing is profound and automatic.

Dr. Kondrot: It sounds like your system is very comprehensive, and you look at many different modalities to help an individual who is suffering from disease or heavy metal poisoning. I wonder if you could give us an example of a patient you treated using some of these methods.

Dr. DeWet: S.S. is a patient I started seeing about 14 years ago in my clinic. He was in congestive heart failure and had ejection fraction of 15 percent. He had suffered at least five heart attacks in his late 30s, which resulted in double bypass surgery. In his 50s, he had to have quadruple bypass. At one point before I started seeing him, he was given fewer than six months to live by the cardiologist who saw him and who did a procedure on him involving the drilling of tiny holes into his heart muscle "to get more blood vessels to grow into the heart muscle." Unfortunately, that didn't work at all and just made him worse. He suffered from a series of other illnesses, including Type 2 diabetes with extreme insulin resistance. He was on over 150 units of insulin total per day and took long-acting insulin. He had a series of other health challenges, including sleep apnea, COPD, severe fluid retention, morbid obesity, chronic low back problems, sciatica, and arthritis in his knees, lower back, shoulders, and neck. He had radiculopathies affecting both arms due to arthritis of the cervical spine causing nerve compression. He had been injured as a paratrooper and broke both ankles after a parachute jump. He later broke his neck while working in the oilfield, but he was not permanently paralyzed and was able to recover from that. He had been diagnosed with over 30 health challenges when he started seeing me and was taking 35 different prescription medications regularly.

We took him in as a patient, and he immediately started EDTA chelation therapy with the disodium magnesium EDTA combined with other standard nutrient ingredients in the IV and followed with hydrogen peroxide IV therapy in a combination called chelox therapy. In addition, he was given IV phosphatidylcholine. He initially completed a series of 20 treatments doing two IVs per week followed by 20 more treatments done weekly. He also did hyperbaric oxygen therapy completing at least 20 treatments over about ten weeks. For his cardiovascular disease, he was treated with a series of supplements, including high dose Coenzyme Q10, omega 3 fatty acids (fish oil), D ribose, L-carnitine, L-arginine, magnesium malate, trimethylglysine combined with methylcobalamine, vitamin B6, an active form of folic acid, proteolytic enzymes, and a series of other supplements for his other health challenges.

He also followed an aggressive detox protocol with a series of ion cleanse foot detoxes, laser energetic detoxification (LED) mentioned earlier in this chapter, and a series of oral detox supplements. These included burbur, parsley, sparga, and pinella (duel action herbal and homeopathic remedies from Nutramedics), Lymph II and Viscum Force from Bioactive Homeopathics, R-lipoic acid, NAC, glutathione, vitamin C, and broad-spectrum vitamin E to facilitate those detox pathways that are responsible for removing metals and other toxins from the body. We also used an oral chelation protocol, including DMSA, zeolite, and chlorella to assist in clearing heavy metals. I also had him get his mercury fillings removed. We had a biological dentist involved in his care.

We also worked on his metabolism. I had him make massive changes to his diet, placing him on a low glycemic index, alkalinizing diet with relatively large amounts of healthy fats. We first had to work on his motivation to make the necessary changes by addressing the underlying conflicts that led to his tendencies to self-sabotage. There were some deep emotional aspects involved that had to be addressed. We know from Recall Healing that the program of diabetes is severe, overwhelming resistance combined with "repugnance" (something stinks in my territory). There were a number of things he had not cleared in his life, including relationship issues ending in divorce and estrangement from his children. We addressed those and other conflicts that had set the stage for his conditions.

The result is that he lost about 50 pounds and achieved massive improvement in his cardiovascular functions. His cardiac ejection fraction improved from 15 percent to 35 percent six months later. During that period, he went from being wheelchair bound to getting rid of his wheelchair six weeks later, feeling a whole lot better, being able to play golf again, and able to participate fully in his own life again. He was able to come off most of his medications, including statins that conventional physicians had placed him on which were contributing to his congestive heart failure. He went from 35 to 7 medications. He still had to take a little bit of a diuretic and some insulin, although we helped him cut his insulin dosage back significantly. At one stage, we had him almost completely off his insulin and all medications. There was great improvement and even full reversal of a number of his health challenges including his sleep apnea. His back pain improved dramatically. His neck pain resolved. There was also a dramatic improvement in his energy and attitude towards his life overall.

Another quick example is L.H., a 63-year-old man when he first started seeing me in 2002. He had had a stroke eight years ago which left him paralyzed in his left arm. On a carotid sonogram done prior to him starting to see me, he had complete occlusion of his right internal carotid artery (RICA) and 70 percent stenosis of the left internal carotid artery (LICA) with ulcerative plaque noted. He had marked financial limitations and was basically only able to afford IV EDTA chelation therapy with disodium magnesium EDTA in long bag form mixed with other nutrients. After ten chelation therapies received twice a week, he had another carotid sonogram done after being seen at a local emergency room after a stressful event for possible transient ischemic attack (TIA) symptoms. Remarkably, his carotid sonogram now showed less than 30 percent stenosis in his LICA with ulcerative plaque resolved. He was also started on some very basic supplements like omega 3 fatty acids, CoQ10, broad-spectrum vitamin E, vitamin C, and magnesium malate. He has done maintenance therapy with IVs once a month since then and continues to do well clinically.

. . . .

Dr. Kondrot: That's an amazing story, and I think it really illustrates the benefits of using multiple modalities and being persistent. It also shows that the course of the illness in most cases is not short-term, and chelation and detoxification are not quick fixes. What can you advise people who are reading this to do right now to improve their health?

Dr. DeWet: There are certain key principles that make healing much more likely to happen. First thing is to help a patient understand that healing is achievable in most instances if they are clear on what they want to achieve, are committed to doing what it takes to heal, and are motivated to take those steps. First, there needs to be a strong desire for healing. They also have to believe that they can heal, that in fact they will heal, and that they deserve to heal. I like to make the point to my patients that there's no such thing as an incurable illness. Even Ebola or rabies have cure rates of at least 50 percent, and most physicians know of patients diagnosed with Stage 4 cancers who have had spontaneous remissions. That's the important thing. It gives people not just hope but a clear vision of what can be accomplished if they get down to business and down to the roots of the illness.

In my book, *Heal Thyself: Transform Your Life, Transform Your Health*, I lay out 18 basic steps critical for optimizing health starting with nutrition and learning what our bodies need in order to heal or stay healthy—understanding that each person is unique. There is no one perfect diet for everyone. By knowing more about yourself, your food sensitivities, your blood type, your disease or health condition, and all of that, you can make a tremendous difference in your own health by consuming what your body needs. That goes for supplementation too.

When people eat right, they tend to feel better, and that makes it easier to continue doing the right thing. I prefer using the term "healthy eating" rather than the term "diet." It's also very important to teach patients how to optimize hydration with the consumption of health promoting fluids including adequate, clean alkaline water. Most people with chronic illnesses are chronically dehydrated. They are also usually too acidic. This can be verified with pH strips and testing one's urine and saliva. Eating much greater amounts of alkalinizing foods versus acid-forming foods can make a tremendous difference in how people feel.

Other critical keys include getting enough sleep. Most of us are sleep deprived. Most of us also don't get enough sun. We actually have entire industries built around keeping the sun off of our skins, at least the rays that are health promoting and that give us the conversion of vitamin D to its active form. Vitamin D3 acts like a hormone in the body. It's critical for healthy bones, healthy immune systems, metabolism and mood control, and for reducing inflammation.

We have them work on detoxification, as explained earlier, including the removal of heavy metals from the body which is critical in order to improve health and overcome disease. Both intravenous and oral chelation methods are extremely helpful in achieving this. For proper detoxification to take place, it is also critical for them to support their primary detox organs, including their gut, liver, kidneys, and lymphatics, for example. I also teach my patients how to reduce their exposure to environmental toxins and toxins in their food and water supply.

I also have them focus on the health of their most important relationships. Toxic relationships contribute greatly to poor health and make it a lot harder to heal, whereas strong vibrant relationships make healing a lot easier to achieve. I remind people how important it is to maintain a good sense of humor and learn to laugh at themselves and even at adversity. The more we laugh, the healthier we tend to be.

Having a clear purpose for one's life—living a purpose-driven life—is also critically important for healing. So is the ability to overcome loss, which is an inevitable part of life. Having a spiritual perspective on life and believing in a higher power has been shown to correlate with better health outcomes. An attitude of gratitude is also critical which is a lot easier to achieve with the use of Recall Healing. This process helps demonstrate that all illnesses are meaningful and purposeful, and the brain's best solution to help ensure short-term survival.

Dr. Ryke Hamer taught us a tremendous amount about the role that conflicts play in the development of disease through his body of work including the evaluation and treatment of over 40,000 cancer patients. He demonstrated that each of them had a significant emotional insult that took place anywhere from two months to two years prior to the development of their cancers. An estimated 93 percent of the patients he saw turned into long-term survivors with most clearing their cancers without any conventional or treatments other than his process involving the discovery and resolution of their disease-causing conflicts. (German New Medicine www.germannewmedicine.ca)

Most importantly, I teach my patients that healing can be and should be fun. By taking a holistic approach, this is achievable, even with life threatening illnesses. Getting healthy also happens to be the most cost-effective medicine, which in this day and age is critical for us to understand.

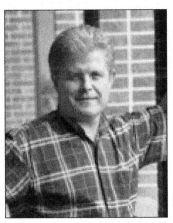

Pieter J. DeWet, MD, MD(H), FAAFP, ABIHM
Quantum Healing Institute
212 Old Grande Blvd., Suite C114
Tyler, TX 75703
903-939-2069
www.Qhiwellness.com

MERCURY MAY BE THE PROBLEM FOR NEARLY EVERYONE

Interview with
Bruce Dooley, MD

I'm excited about the healing work helping people with chronic health problems and helping them function naturally, often without the need for prescription medication or surgery. For the past 15 years, I've been using the latest advances in the field of integrative medicine to help a wide range of people, from those desiring prevention and more energy to those with the most debilitating illnesses.

For nearly a decade, I treated colds and flus, sutured lacerations, set broken bones, counseled people with cholesterol and weight problems, responded to the drama of chest pains, and offered advice and comfort when life's stresses literally made patients sick. After treating thousands of patients, the same question kept nagging at me: Why are so many people getting sick and how can I help them prevent it?

I was no longer satisfied providing prescription medications and surgery to patients with chronic illnesses since they don't CURE the condition but merely suppress the symptoms. I realized that symptoms such as fatigue and poor vitality are warning signs of a system out of balance, yet nothing from my medical school training—no prescription medication or surgery—would help restore that balance. I began studying with healers who used nutrition, mind-body medicine, chiropractic, acupuncture, herbology, ho-

meopathy, magnet therapy, bodywork, and other healing arts. Since then, I've treated over 30,000 patients with integrative medicine for arteriosclerosis, heavy metal toxicity, memory problems, fatigue, autoimmune disorders, and other chronic diseases.

In 2001, I began routinely screening and treating patients for the presence of mercury, one of the most toxic substances known to man. It is my vision to see the world's population mercury free and healthy. As a physician, my mission is to help restore people's health, energy, and reason for living by offering education, conversation, and science-based alternatives to surgery and prescription medications.

1. **Chelation is one of the most, if not the most, effective anti-aging therapies.**

2. **In disease medicine, doctors are trained to be at the bottom of the cliff diagnosing the crash.**

3. **Chelation will increase blood vessel elasticity and turn the clock back 15 to 20 years.**

. . . .

Dr. Kondrot: Tell us a little bit about your medical training and background.

Dr. Dooley: I'm conventionally trained. I received my bachelor's in Philadelphia, my master's in immunology at Villanova, and my MD at Thomas Jefferson in Philadelphia. I trained allopathically and went on to do emergency medicine. Along the way, I built two urgent care centers, one in Park City, Utah, and one in Fort Lauderdale, Florida. Eventually I focused on Fort Lauderdale.

Somewhere along the line in my urgent care walk-in center, around 1990, a patient told me that his life had been saved by this therapy called EDTA chelation. I had known that EDTA was used for lead, but I couldn't figure out what the heck he was talking about. He told me he read a book called *Bypassing Bypass* by Elmer Cranton, a Harvard-trained MD in West Virginia who had 20 years of experience in chelation. I bought the book and started reading it, and I was amazed. I said, "This guy can't be making this up.

I attended a training session in ACAM, the American College for Advancement in Medicine, where I eventually became a director. I quietly put a couple of chairs in the back of my urgent walk-in care center in Fort Lauderdale. It was very quietly done because, back in those times, this was really voodoo stuff. I began to take patients I thought could use chelation, people with angina, claudication pain in the legs, erectile dysfunction, memory issues, and high blood pressure. I was amazed at the results. They were literally shocking beyond belief. One guy, an 83-year-old, went from totally deaf to totally hearing again. He didn't need his hearing aids by the tenth treatment. That freaked me out. I was amazed a lot in the beginning. People's blood pressure went down so fast you had to take them off the medicine because they'd get hypotensive. All these things now, after 4,000 patients, have become kind of standard.

I said, "This is too good to do in the back room of my office." I decided to open up dedicated centers in Fort Lauderdale and Naples, Florida, where we had 20-plus recliner chairs, and we were committed to infusion therapy. It was mostly magnesium EDTA chelation therapy but also high-dose vitamin C, nutritional IVs and things like that. Between the two centers, I was chelating 100 patients a day. I was arguably one of the biggest chelating docs at the time. I was getting tremendous results and zero negative side effects. From my own experience, there was 85 percent improvement. That 85 percent is the same number that keeps coming up in Terry Chappell's meta-analysis of 22,000 patients that was done with objective instrument testing of EDTA chelation. I went on to teaching chelation to other doctors and lecturing about it extensively. I believe it is one of the most, if not the most, effective anti-aging therapies known.

Then I got very involved with mercury. As a matter of course, all my patients who wanted chelation were required to go through a combined EDTA and DMPS provocative testing of heavy metals through Doctor's Data lab. I began to see a significant number of people with mercury. This really began to change my life, especially since my father, a brilliant physician and father of eight, died of dementia at 69. He had a mouthful of mercury and ate fish every Friday as a good Catholic. I really believe his dementia was mercury associated. It's a personal story for me.

Mercury, which is an area I really want to talk about, is toxic at any level. That's from the World Health Organization. It is responsible for pan systemic involvement in just about every organ system, enzyme pathway, and mitochondrial function.

Dr. Kondrot: You were really shocked when you saw how effective chelation can be when treating chronic disease. Of course, that's the way I felt when I began using it for eye disease. Why do you think the public is not more aware of these therapies? What's the biggest stumbling block?

Dr. Dooley: Let me finish this story. I left the country. I wasn't going to come back. I got pulled back into the country by accident, just at the time the TACT trial was being announced by Dr. Gervasio Lamas. I bought the live feed for that November 3, 2012, American Heart Association delivery. It was interesting that you could hear a pin drop in that room. It's almost like there was a shock that ran through the cardiologists. "Oh, my gosh, they've done it."

Dr. Kondrot: Tell us a little more about that. Some of the people out there are not familiar with the TACT study.

Dr. Dooley: EDTA chelation therapy began in the '60s; Norm Clarke discovered its vascular effect by accident while he was chelating lead-toxic battery workers with EDTA. He began to see all of these vascular improvements. He and a bunch of physicians at the Henry Ford Hospital in Detroit began to use EDTA for vascular conditions, and they were getting profound improvements in the 85 percent area.

Abbott Labs owned the patent on EDTA for lead, and they got very excited. They said, "This is a secondary application. It could be unbelievable." They launched into a program of making applications to the FDA for secondary approval. Then the patent expired, right in the middle of their application. No one is going to do a millions-of-dollars study on a non-patentable drug, so for the next 50 years, this association formed out of Norm Clarke and a small group called the American Preventics. Jim Frackelton was one of the members. They developed protocols. They trained more and more doctors. They started doing this, and it grew.

This therapy grew in the face of another therapy that the bean counters at the hospitals loved much more. That was the bypass surgery pioneered by Denton Cooley in Houston, and later the stents for handling coronary vessel disease.

This is what happened to a therapy that was 100 percent safe and almost 85 percent effective. It was completely washed down the tubes because it was not expensive and, in my experience, removed potential patients from the $200,000 bypasses at the time and later from the stents market. My sense right now is that 95 percent of the patients who came to me and were told that they had to have a stent or bypass and were brave enough to get off the table and get a second opinion never had to go back for a stent or bypass.

One cardiologist who was politically powerful tried to stop chelations through the Board of Medicine in Florida. We had a march of 1,000 patients in Tampa. Chelation therapy has been protected in Florida after that event. We actually got a law passed. The statute passed in the Florida legislature in 2001 with the backing of the Hilton family. It protects us using any therapies with informed consent. I'm going to investigate much more about what we can actually do here in Florida with that statute.

Here's the situation. The patients interested in chelation would invariably go to their cardiologist and ask, "What do you think about this?" They would be told by the cardiologist most of the time that it was voodoo and/or quackery, and/or they would say, "Forget about it. You're wasting your money." Some of them would say, "It can't hurt you, but there's no proof." They all basically fell back on saying that there's no hard evidence of the double-blind, placebo-controlled type.

We grew organically. Patients would come in because they saw what happened to their colleague, family member, or friend. They would see these results and want them. They were willing to pay out of pocket because it's not reimbursable by insurance. They were willing to do the time in the chair, as we call it. You have to do the time in the chair.

For the TACT trial, we ended up going to the complementary and alternative medicine wing of the NIH. The initial application was turned down by the board that studied this, mostly made up of cardiologists. I got the records of their meeting by the Freedom of Information Act and passed it around to people because it was startling what they were saying about chelation. The most startling statement was when one of the cardiologists said, "What really worries me is 'what if it's true? What if it works?'" That was a statement that I have on tape.

They canned it the first time but passed it the second time. It was a $35 million seven-year multi-center study involving 1,700 enrollees. All needed to have a prior MI (myocardial infarction: heart attack). It was a very difficult recruitment because the subjects had a 50/50 chance of spending hundreds of hours in the chair and getting placebo. Unlike a placebo pill, this was a difficult requirement.

It lasted nearly a decade, and it was announced in 2012 and published in *JAMA*. The next year, Dr. Lamas surprised us all because we didn't know he had looked at the diabetic cohort subsection of the trial, and the study showed a 50 percent improvement in the treated diabetic patients over the diabetic patients who took placebo—and with zero risk. There were two big questions they wanted to answer. Was it safe? Yes. Was it effective? Yes. That was published.

. . . .

Dr. Kondrot: Maybe you could explain exactly how they define improvement.

Dr. Dooley: The really sad thing about this study is that they failed to extend the endpoints. They only looked at four endpoints. Did the person need to have another bypass? Did they need to have restenting? Did they have another heart attack? Did they die? Based on those four endpoints, there was a statistically significant improvement over the placebo in all four. However, things such as claudication pain, walking distance, angina pain, blood pressure, arterial elasticity, calcium scoring, and carotid stenosis could have been looked at, but they weren't. We have to put up with the way it was. The comment at the end of that 2012 announcement by Dr. Lamas was, "That's very well and good, but we can't recommend it clinically yet. More studies are needed." What I'm trying to do now is outcome studies with local cardiologists.

. . . .

Dr. Kondrot: If you had to get a message out to the public, what is that message?

Dr. Dooley: The important message to the public is that lifestyles involving smoking, high stress levels, and high levels of heavy metal promote free radical oxidative stresses on the body. One of the major things to understand is that when arteries are bombarded by heavy metal and all these other free radical insulters, the end result is a hardening of the arteries, a process called arteriosclerosis. It's not necessarily atherosclerosis. The actual elasticity of the arteries begins to be diminished. (Editor's Note: Atherosclerosis is a specific form of arteriosclerosis in which an artery wall thickens as a result of invasion and accumulation of white blood cells.)

That's a very interesting thing because there's a fluid flow law called Poiseuille's Law. When you diminish the diameter of a pipe carrying fluid by 15 percent, you actually halve the flow. The inverse of every law has to be true too. When you increase a pipe by 15 percent, you double the flow. Just like a car engine needs fuel and gets rid of exhaust, our mitochondria need oxygen fuel and to get rid of exhaust. There's only one system in the body that does that. It's the circulatory system. If Poiseuille's Law is in effect, and it is, then with chronological and biological aging, at the arterial level you begin to see diminished performance. What we call the "dwindles" begins to happen in people. They begin to manifest symptoms of poor mitochondrial function, fatigue, memory issues, erectile issues, and other issues you can clearly associate with the heart. These conditions are given a lot of names and there are a lot of medicines for them.

The point is that I encourage people to be proactive. We take care of our cars better than we take care of ourselves. In disease care medicine, the doctors are trained to be at the bottom of the cliff diagnosing the crash. The patients are told to wait around until something breaks. Then go to the doctor. That's when the system starts making money. But we are proactive doctors, and patients need to be proactive too.

What I am trying to tell people is to think about being ahead of the equation and not necessarily wait for something to happen. Try to think about doing therapy that will increase blood vessel elasticity by 15 to 20 years with a 20-treatment chelation program. That's my estimate of what people need. You actually turn the clock back 15 to 20 years on the arterial side.

We were taught at medical school about essential hypertension. I love that. What does that mean? It means you need to have it? They blew that by us in pathology. I tell patients, "You go in year after year to get a physical by your doctor. When you're around 45 or 50, there's a double take, and your doctor says, 'You have hypertension. You need to be on medicine the rest of your life.'" That's it.

When I talk to groups of people in the public, I say that if you went in with a pain in your side and the doctor said, "Take these pills for the rest of your life and don't worry about the pain," you'd ask, "What's causing the pain?" Nobody seems to say, "Last year my blood pressure was fine, but now I need to be on medicine for the rest of my life. What happened in between?" The doctor would then scratch his head and say, "We call it essential hypertension." That's not an answer. The answer is that Poiseuille's Law starts kicking in as the elasticity threshold is hit, and then the pressures go up. That's why, with almost 90 percent certainty, people who do chelation therapy are able to get off their blood pressure medicines. If they don't, they often will find it's due to renal stenosis.

. . . .

Dr. Kondrot: All doctors have a unique approach. We hear about IV chelation, rectal chelation, and oral chelation. What is your unique approach?

Dr. Dooley: I had an epiphany back in the early 2000s. I began to see that all of this mercury was showing up in people when I tested them, but I knew EDTA did not bind to chelate mercury. It hit me, very sadly, with a case of a guy named Bob Director who was owner of Director Ganahl Boatyard. He had done about 50 chelations. He was a big, strapping 80-year-old guy. He was taking Tae Kwon Do. He sailed his 70-foot boat to Norway single-handedly. He's Norwegian. He was that kind of guy.

One day he came in and told me he had pancreatic cancer. I said, "Oh, my God, Bob." The one thing we didn't look at—because I wasn't doing it at that time—was a multi-metal challenge, so I did one on him. I used Doctor's Data lab using DMPS and EDTA. Two days later, he died. The day I went to his funeral, his mercury report came back from Doctor's Data at 900. The edge of the page is 20, so 900 is almost 45 times off the page. It turned out that in the old days they used mercuric oxide as the antifouling paint on boats because nothing could grow on this poison, which is second only to plutonium in toxicity. He must have been inhaling the sand that was in his boatyard for all those years and accumulated this massive amount of mercury, which I believe was the causal agent for his pancreatic cancer.

I vowed then and there that no one was going to get past me without testing for mercury. If they were high and I'm not getting it out with EDTA, as obviously was true in this case, I would do my job as a physician and do the best for my patients. Off I went testing everyone. DMPS (dimercapto propane sulfonic acid) is an amazing chelator. It's been around for 50 or 60 years. It was discovered in Russia. In fact, our DMPS comes from Russia because it's the purest. It is essentially as nontoxic as it can be. It's one of the safest chemicals and one of the most studied. Germany has a 1,000-page monograph about it. I began to realize that I was not doing my job if I didn't do heavy metal testing and rule out mercury because mercury is probably the most toxic metal.

. . . .

Dr. Kondrot: What do you feel is the best way to test for mercury?

Dr. Dooley: David Quig from Doctor's Data is quite an expert on this. Hair, blood, and random urine are not good for testing. Blood samples are always negative for heavy metals, particularly mercury.

. . . .

Dr. Kondrot: I think we have to emphasize that. Typically, if a patient goes to a traditional Western doctor, he'll do a blood and urine and say, "It's garbage. You don't have heavy metals in your body. Why are you getting chelation?" I think it is critical for people to understand why they need a challenge test?

Dr. Dooley: Let me give you an example. I spoke in front of two sessions, a year apart, of 1,200 people each time. This was the first large cohort of normal people ever in history using provoked urine challenge. It was 1,200 people. I'll tell you in a minute what happened there. One of the attendees to this fitness conference was a female dentist in her 50s. She contacted me and said, "I think I'm toxic with mercury." It's terrible what has happened to dentists. They're so polluted. She went to her regular doctor and said, "I'm a dentist. I'm exposed to mercury. I think mercury toxicity may be behind all these neurological and emotional symptoms I'm having." He said it was a bunch of baloney, but she forced him to take a blood test, which of course was negative. He said, "Ha, ha. Do you see what I mean?" When she did the provoked urine challenge with me, it was two or three times off the page.

This has been a pattern that repeats itself all the time. If people do non-provoked urine challenges and send in pre-provocation testing, which I gave up on because it's just an extra expense, all of them are pretty much negative. There's nothing coming out in the random urine because if it's not in the blood, it's not going to be in the urine or get into the hair. You have to think about this for a second. Metals are in the tissues. Just sticking a needle in somebody's arm doesn't mean they're going to say, "We're here." You have to physically grab the metals with a chelating agent. Then it pulls them into the blood and urine, and you can collect the urine sample and get a spectroscopic analysis by an excellent lab like Doctor's Data to prove that the tissues are loaded with metals.

· ·

Dr. Kondrot: Please go over exactly how you recommend the challenge test be done?

Dr. Dooley: DMPS is 50 percent to 60 percent absorbed orally. Therefore, it makes no sense to give an IV because there can be some serious outcomes from IV. I'm telling doctors now, "Don't use IV. Just use the oral DMPS in the provocation test." Five-hundred milligrams for most people does just fine. It's taken on an empty stomach after the morning void. You can eat 20 minutes after it clears the stomach. Then you collect urine for the next three hours. Only collect the three hours' worth because that's going to show you the highest concentration. Then you pour a sample and send it off. All of this is included in the Doctor's Data collections kit. You receive a very nice, colored, detailed analysis.

People ask, "What do I do when the value is high?" We simply suggest they get on an oral program of DMPS with a good mineral supplementation and something that upregulates the production of glutathione because the significant reduction in glutathione and selenium by mercury contributes a lot to the oncogenic (tumor producing) effect of mercury. It takes two glutathione to remove every atom of mercury. If you have amalgams, they're putting off millions of atoms of mercury every day. You're effectively using up doubles of millions of molecules of glutathione. It takes two selenium atoms for every mercury atom, so it turns into mercuric selenide. You're using up selenium and glutathione, two no-nos when it comes to preserving the immune system. People with high mercury readings are going to show significant glutathione reduction and selenium reduction. You're going to see a lowered white blood count many times, a nice little jewel that physicians need to know about. When they see a low white count and there's no sign of infection, it's almost always mercury or lead.

Lead and mercury together create a synergistic explosion. One plus one can equal 100 as far as neurotoxicity. It's not one plus one equals two. We're seeing a lot of lead come out of people who have lived in big cities when there was leaded gasoline—New York, north Jersey, and Chicago. You don't see a lot of lead in people who lived out in the country.

. . . .

Dr. Kondrot: I think it's essential that you take a glutathione and selenium supplement. How do you incorporate that in your protocol? Let's talk about some of your favorite products and your protocol.

Dr. Dooley: I don't want this to be a commercialization, but the only product I and many others now use is a product called MercOut. It has the morning formula containing upregulators to glutathione production in your body and the minerals. Then there's the nighttime formula of DMPS. It's a 30-day treatment program that's been in effect for seven or eight years with over 5,000 people. It's been very safe and very well tolerated by most people. I do that. Often they need to have more than a 30-day treatment, so we go on to 60 or 90 days and then retest them, depending on where their initial report comes. We get about a 15-point lowering in mercury with each 30-day program.

That leads to the next thing about sequestration. Mercury and lead tend to sequester themselves deeply into the deeper tissues. There is a problem with the provoked test. It's the gold standard in our case until somebody invents a scanner, like with a calcium scoring device, and we can get an exact count of mercury and lead in the body. Wouldn't that be nice?

Often we give both DMPS and EDTA if patients want to get the best challenge. We will give the IV EDTA and the oral together. Those chelators that they're circulating around can only grab on to what they can grab on to. In many cases, if there's a lot of mercury and lead, the chelating compound is completely tied up, and there's actually more there than what is revealed.

Even though you get a quantitative number from Doctor's Data, that's something that has to be understood in the context of what I'm saying. A lot of times people will do chelation for mercury or lead, and the numbers will come down or they won't. I have a case where an eight-year-old boy and his father have taken eight treatments of MercOut and continue to have high levels. We can't figure that out. But most people see their mercury levels go down. If they don't have an ongoing source of contamination, such as the amalgams, a lot of times they'll come back a year later and their number will have risen again, but not so much. It comes out of the bone and the deeper tissue. Then we tell them to do another MercOut. Personally, I do one 30-day program a year anyway just because I want to keep cleaning myself out.

· ·

Dr. Kondrot: When someone demonstrates an extremely high level of mercury, there are certain things you think of. Do they have mercury amalgams? Have they accumulated mercury in their bones? What other factors do you think people should look for when they have an extremely high level of mercury? How should they be evaluated?

Dr. Dooley: Once you've gotten a test score back with high mercury, you might want to check blood levels of glutathione. I don't do that routinely. I just go on the assumption that they need glutathione and selenium. The symptomatology changes as they're getting rid of mercury is the powerful thing. They see symptoms reduce, no matter what they might be. Under the emotions, we have rage, anger, depression, mood swings, anxiety, irritability, brain fog, and dementia. I've seen remarkable turnarounds in dementia that I think is way over-diagnosed as being Alzheimer's. Organic brain syndrome means basically that the brain requires a lot of oxygen and it's not getting it anymore, so their brain is struggling along and not doing a good job.

You see arrhythmias go away. The Frustaci study is a very important study. In 1999 in Rome, a group of cardiologists took 13 people with failing hearts. They published this in the *American Journal of Cardiology*. While these 13 people were waiting for a heart transplant, they decided to do something pretty extraordinary. They did myocardial biopsies for heavy metals. They also took biopsies from each person's skeletal muscle too, the same side, and sent them in for analysis. The report was astonishing to us in the heavy metal toxicology field. On average, for these 13 patients, there was 22,000 times more mercury in the heart muscle than in the thigh muscle of the same person. There were thousands of times more cadmium in the heart muscle and thousands of times more lead. Every single toxic metal that they studied was massively elevated in the heart.

What is mercury? It is one of the most potent neurotoxins. What is the heart? Outside of the brain, it is one of the biggest nerve bundles. If you super concentrate mercury in the heart muscle, what's going to start happening to the heart? These were failing hearts. Upstream, it's arrhythmias. It's going to affect the electrical patterns of the heart. If you chelate patients with arrhythmias with DMPS and EDTA for lead and mercury, the arrhythmias will go away. It's the same with blood pressure.

Back to my story. When we tested the 1,200 healthy people ages 17 to 70 at these two fitness talks I gave, using Doctor's Data, I was shocked. I had no idea what to expect. We handed out mirrors to everybody and had them count their amalgams. Then we went through a raise of hands. How many had six, five, four, three, or two? How many people have never had any amalgams? About five percent of people in the room—the younger ones—had never had amalgams. When our results came in, 75 percent of the 1,200 patients were in the red zone for mercury. Twenty percent were in the yellow zone. Only five percent were in the green zone. I kicked myself for not getting the names of people who had never had amalgams to correlate, but I'm sure that's what it was. The people who never had amalgams were most likely the ones in the green zone. That was pretty cool.

If you extrapolate to how many millions of people in the United States in a certain age range had these poisons planted in their heads, we're talking about a massive number of people with mercury toxicity.

It's been a really wild ride for me. I have a lot of scars on my back from arrows shot at me, but I think it's becoming more and more acceptable to the public and, hopefully, through doctors that they should really test themselves.

· ·

Dr. Kondrot: If there were a takeaway you could give people who read this chapter, what would that be?

Dr. Dooley: If you have amalgams, you have been contaminated by mercury. My suggestion is not to go running out and get the amalgams removed right away. You could get really toxic by doing that. It's a 4,000 fold increase in your stored mercury level if not done properly. We actually give people DMPS before, during, and after amalgam removal so they can protect themselves to some extent.

If you have any of the symptomologies—and we haven't even gone through the list of symptoms known to be caused by mercury—and you're suspicious of it, get testing done. If your level is high and you do have a pathology that is likely associated with mercury, do an oral detoxification. A combination of EDTA and DMPS is the best. Then and only then, can you safely get those amalgams removed.

I tell medical students and doctors that they need to do an amalgam history. When they're doing a history, they need to look in the mouth, not just at the tonsils, uvula, and tongue. If there are amalgams, make note of how many there are. If there are amalgams opposed to another metal, like gold, then you have a really bad situation. That's called the Oral Galvanic Effect, and you get a much higher release of the metals of the amalgam. If you're an older person and you have no amalgams, recall when the amalgams were removed. Many times, you'll find it coincides with the onset of your health issues. It was the trigger that made you fall off the cliff.

Have the amalgams removed and continue on a yearly basis to look at how your mercury and lead are doing because they will continue to come out of the tissues. If you want to sweep it again, do so. It may take five years of doing this once a year to finally get cleaned up. Metals are not meant to be removed aggressively. My theory is that they should be removed slowly. The detox pathways need to be opened.

It helps to get Myers' cocktails or high dose IV vitamin C, which itself is a chelator along with IV glutathione. That's a really helpful process. You can now take oral glutathione in a form which is well-absorbed. There's selenium, of course, too. These are my suggestions. It's not really hard to do, but it is vital to do it.

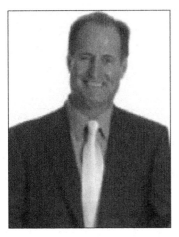

Bruce Dooley, MD
Advanced Natural Medicine
240 W. Indiantown Rd. #102
Jupiter, FL 33458
www.drdooley.com
561-744-2724

POISONED PLANET, POISONED PEOPLE: DETOXIFY DAILY

Interview with
Garry F. Gordon, MD, DO, MD(H)

Garry F. Gordon, MD, DO, MD(H), received his Doctor of Osteopathy in 1958 from the Chicago College of Osteopathy in Illinois. He received his honorary MD degree from the University of California Irvine in 1962 and completed his radiology residency from Mt. Zion in San Francisco, California in 1964. For many years, he was the medical director of Mineral Lab in Hayward, California, a leading laboratory for trace mineral analysis worldwide.

Dr. Gordon served on the Board of Homeopathic Medical Examiners for Arizona and is co-founder of the American College for Advancement in Medicine (ACAM). He is the founder/president of the International College of Advanced Longevity Medicine (ICALM) and board member of International Oxidative Medicine Association (IOMA).

With Morton Walker, DPM, Dr. Gordon co-authored The Chelation Answer. *He is advisor to the American Board of Chelation Therapy and past instructor and examiner for all chelation physicians. He is responsible for Peer Review for Chelation Therapy in the State of Arizona.*

As an internationally recognized expert on chelation therapy, Dr. Gordon is now attempting to establish standards for the proper use of oral and intravenous chelation therapy as an adjunct therapy for all diseases. He lectures extensively on the subject, "The End of Bypass Surgery Is in Sight."

Currently, Dr. Gordon is a consultant for various supplement companies. He is responsible for the design of many supplements, which are widely used by alternative health practitioners around the world.

1. **We all need a lifetime detoxification program.**

2. **I have not heard of any patient who had a fatal heart attack or stroke if they consistently followed my chelation protocol.**

3. **There is a direct correlation between toxic chemicals and the increase in ADD, autism, dyslexia, and oppositional behavior disorder.**

4. **Chelated parents produce healthy babies. Infants are now born with 300 toxins in their bodies, passed on from the mother.**

. . . .

Dr. Kondrot: Please tell us about your medical training and how you became interested in chelation and other vital detox methods.

Dr. Gordon: I am the son of a gifted osteopathic physician, and I decided by age nine that I wanted to be a physician. I applied to the Osteopathic College when I was about 14 years old to let them know I was coming and to please save me a place. I studied at the University of Wisconsin and the University of Chicago. Then I received my DO degree in 1958 from what was then the Chicago College of Osteopathy. After graduation, I did my internship in Boston and then began practicing in a 24-hour emergency medical center in California.

After a few years there, I decided to become a radiologist. A year later, I discovered chelation therapy due to a major health problem involving my heart. For me, this was a miracle. I had never been strong and had been unable to go up a flight of stairs without becoming seriously short of breath for most of my life.

When I was a young boy, I developed many dental cavities related to the various health problems I had had from birth. They included recurring high fevers, stuttering, disabling fatigue, constant headaches, etc. When my father took me to a dentist, he ended up filling almost every tooth with amalgam, which contains a lot of mercury. Sometime later, when I was even more ill, my father took me to another dentist who claimed that what the last dentist had done was improper. He took out all my fillings and replaced them— using no precautions—so I was breathing all those mercury fumes. I wound up becoming very ill and almost unable to stay awake. That condition lasted a long time. No one recognized that I had been poisoned; we were simply told I had narcolepsy.

Today, there are better-informed physicians involved in environmental medicine who would correctly diagnose my problem as mercury poisoning. We finally figured that out many years later, and it has required years of intravenous and oral chelation therapy for me to recover, and finally, at age 80, enjoy good health. Those personal events have led me, in my 56 years of medical practice, to focus on the epidemic of generally undiagnosed heavy metal toxicity, which is rampant today. Heavy metals are ubiquitous and are able to produce almost any symptom. Yet, they are still largely ignored by most physicians who see patients every day whose lives could be improved dramatically if they undertook a program of long-term chelation-based detoxification.

Today, I teach that some form of daily detoxification is important for everyone. Chelation is a passion with me. Before I discovered intravenous chelation, I was so sick and toxic that I closed my medical office because I could not walk from room to room without becoming extremely fatigued. However, after my first eight IV chelation sessions, I was able, for the first time in my life, to jog up the side of a very steep mountain while wearing out my two-year-old Irish setter.

Chelation therapy was finally beginning to help my body get the toxins like lead and mercury out. Since then I have been a strong advocate for the unrecognized need for all of us to get the lead and other toxins out, even if that takes years.

Detoxification is essential if we hope to reach our maximum intended useful life span.

. . . .

Dr. Kondrot: You were one of the founding fathers of one of the organizations that taught physicians how to do chelation, the American College for Advancement in Medicine. How have things evolved over the years in terms of approaches to chelation? What are the important things the public needs to know about chelation and detox?

Dr. Gordon: The public needs to know that every one of us should be on a detox program, ideally even before we even choose a partner to have a baby. The toxins from the mother are being concentrated in the baby. The placenta is not the protective barrier we once thought it was. Any chemicals or toxins that are absorbed into the mother's body and bloodstream get passed through the umbilical cord into her child. The net result is that today we are all averaging at least 1,000 to 2,000 times more lead in our bones than anyone who lived before the industrial age on Earth—700 years ago. In that short span of a few hundred years, our bodies have been unable to adapt to these levels of lead and mercury. I believe that we cannot enjoy optimal health and longevity unless we learn about our absolute need for daily, lifetime detoxification. This can be achieved with natural products like vitamin C if taken in 8000 mg a day doses, also garlic, and some of the other oral chelators.

There are amazing natural detoxifiers available that include mineral zeolite clay, humic and fulvic acids, oral calcium EDTA, and many other useful compounds. I always include EDTA in my oral and intravenous chelation programs. EDTA stands for ethylenediamine tetraacetic acid. Note that vinegar is acetic acid.

We now recognize that the level of lead in our bones is in equilibrium with our brain and kidneys, and bones require 15 years to remodel and become new, so there is no overnight program that can resolve our lead toxicity, and there is no safe level of lead in bones as it will always migrate elsewhere in our body.

Chelation therapy can now be oral, or short five-minute IV pushes, or the standard we started with, requiring three hours, and/or even included in bath water. Chelation therapy with magnesium, calcium, or Disodium EDTA, has been shown to improve conditions contributing to arterial stiffness, pulse wave velocity, central blood pressure, and endothelial function. Improving these significantly lowers cardiovascular risks. The $31 million TACT Trial to Assess Chelation Therapy showed the best results in reducing death was in diabetics. So chelation research today has moved far beyond the earlier focus on heart disease, as getting the toxins out clearly involves every aspect of our mental and physical health. A treatment that was once considered useful only for lead workers now has far broader indications. By the time people learn that their poor health is related to toxins, they may want to consider a more concentrated program using both oral and some form of intravenous chelation. Even a single IV chelation can provide benefit depending on the clinical condition, the toxins present, and the chelators used.

We all have numerous health problems today. We think we're just tired or getting forgetful because we are aging, and that's supposed to be normal. We have chest pains and headaches. The list goes on. Whatever your health complaint, your doctor will most likely prescribe some drug or other chemical since most physicians have studied only the pharmaceutical approach. If you want advanced medical care, you need to see a doctor who has an interest in environmental medicine. In the long run, that approach will save you a lot of money, give you a better quality of health, and add years to your life. My experience has shown me that there is no condition—whether you're depressed or you just can't walk around the block anymore or have cancer—that will not benefit from a good chelation program. You can begin to feel well rapidly, because the oral program I have developed can neutralize the toxins so the body can function almost as well as though the toxins were already gone.

Chelation has such broad applications that it almost sounds like a panacea. Scientists hate that idea. Something that cures everything must be imaginary. It seems too good to be true, but it really works. We change lives every day around the world. Tests for heavy metals help determine the level of toxicity, but even when the levels are within the "normal" range, you are not safe. There is no safe level for lead and mercury. Not one of us is reaching our intellectual or full energy capacity because we have toxins in our water, food, and air that clearly adversely affect every part of our lives, including how long and how well we'll live.

Dr. Kondrot: Since you've been in the business of chelation and detoxifying and helping patients achieve their maximum health, you've seen a lot of products and approaches come and go. I wonder if you could share your unique approach when you evaluate a patient, what you recommend, and which products you prefer that they use.

Dr. Gordon: To improve your health, I do not need to know the exact name of your infection. Most infections can be safely treated with a comprehensive oxidative treatment program, particularly when combined with lifetime detoxification. Expensive toxic antibiotics seldom provide any lasting benefit as resistance develops, and the drugs are too toxic or expensive to continue treatment.

But as helpful as blood, urine, and hair testing has been, there are many people with impaired ability to excrete heavy metals so these tests are not perfect. The autistic child may not show any elevated levels of metals, in hair, blood, or urine because of an inability of their cells to detoxify. As a result, the doctor says, "It has nothing to do with toxicity," and couldn't be more wrong. As a matter of fact, researchers at Harvard and Mt. Sinai have recently revealed a direct correlation between toxic chemicals and the pandemic in the neurobehavioral disorders of ADD, autism, dyslexia, oppositional behavior disorder, and many others. Lead and mercury are the first two on their list.

Urine and hair tests help many on their road to recovery because they can help identify those with excess lead, mercury, or cadmium and also identify a deficiency of useful minerals such as zinc and magnesium. Autopsy findings reveal that nearly everyone has had high bone lead levels in the past 100 years, and that means they could have been healthier with chelation. The data we now have strongly suggests that no one on the planet today is living as long or as healthy as they would if they had been lucky enough to be born from chelated parents. The father contributes to the child's loss of health through toxicity that leads to less-than-healthy sperm. Average sperm counts in the past 50 years have dropped from 140 million to just 40 million.

We have poisoned our nest, but now we have the ability to learn and deal with the problem since there are many natural substances available to help us chelate and detoxify. The simplest thing I suggest is to do what Linus Pauling taught us. He was a proponent of vitamin C. If you take 4,000 milligrams of vitamin C twice per day, every day, you are going to have eight grams of vitamin C circulating through your system. Vitamin C is a natural chelator, and although that is only half of the 16+ grams that Linus Pauling took, even eight grams daily is highly beneficial particularly the BioEnRGy C form which provides tremendous benefits. Some may laugh at this and say, "But the vitamin C is going out in the urine." Yes, this is true. That is one of its beneficial mechanisms. When vitamin C goes out, it grabs toxins and carries them out too. This lowers the total body-burden of toxins and poisons that we all carry around and that our babies are being born with today.

Do we know this to be a fact? Yes. Every child born averages at least twice the level of lead and mercury that was in the mother's body. The Environmental Working Group study called Ten Americans proved this. Testing the blood from the umbilical cords of infants showed they were born with some 287 various toxins in their bodies—toxins passed on from the mother. Are we going to get to the point that responsible mothers detox before they decide they're going to have a baby? Yes, I believe with the incidence of autism continuing to rise, parents will begin to understand the need for detoxing long before and during the pregnancy. Fortunately, we are able to restore sick people, as was demonstrated in my personal case, to an amazing level of health by helping them get the lead, mercury, cadmium, and other toxins out and putting in all the vital nutrients so often missing in our diet.

Environmental medicine should be on the front pages of the newspaper every day. We're seeing a lot of concern about what electricity is going to cost if the plants build special filters to scrub the mercury from the exhaust. We always have this tradeoff. What is the cost and what is the benefit? If people knew what health problems we all suffer due to lead and mercury, they would prefer to conserve energy and pay the higher price for clean energy.

I'm a doctor who believes that our bodies were designed to live at least to 120 years. I am now 80 years of age, and, at this point in life, I am enjoying better health than I had when much younger. I'm finally rid of most of the fatigue, heart pain, angina, headaches, and back pain that I suffered with as a young man. Many of the health issues I struggled with for years are gone now because I searched for answers and made the effort to follow my program. I've taken a lot of IV treatments and oral supplements in order to be able to say that, but it is worth it.

. . . .

Dr. Kondrot: Please tell us the steps you take when you see a patient you suspect has toxins or heavy metal poisoning.

Dr. Gordon: I do lab tests, and I like to also have a provoked urine specimen. That is where the patient gets an intravenous or oral chelation dose that causes the body to excrete heavy metals rapidly. The urine is then analyzed so we know what toxins we are dealing with. I want everyone to be aware of what healthful activities we need to be doing, including diet and exercise, but also that there are special things we can do for our bodies. We need to get more fiber, the right greens, zeolite, oral vitamin C, etc., every day. I really like bathing in things like EDTA, zeolite, Epsom salts, and even in oxidative agents like Clorox. I like to have people exercising while breathing oxygen and have people consuming ASEA water for the redox signaling molecules they have been able to stabilize. I am a strong advocate of sweating and far infrared (FIR) saunas, and it is especially beneficial to combine the FIR sauna with ozone therapy, which is one of the best detox methods to rid the body of PCBs, pesticides, and other chemicals. I like to add energy medicine like microcurrent, intranasal laser, and pulsed electromagnetic devices such as PEMF. These can help provide the body with the extra energy it needs to help pump out toxins. There is a need today for detox centers where these methods and even special bathing water will be available.

My personal protocol, including all the supplements that I take on a daily basis, can be found on my website under the heading of "protocols." I also have protocols there for how I treat cancer, heart disease, fibromyalgia, and autoimmune system diseases, and my comprehensive F.I.G.H.T. for Your Health program.

Also on my website is a comprehensive list of 507 clinical published references showing the effectiveness of oral EDTA. Because oral EDTA is not so wellabsorbed, many doctors dismiss it without recognizing its amazing benefits. If they read the abstracts on my website, I believe that they will have to admit they were wrong and add oral EDTA to any detox program they are using.

My health-promoting program also deals with the chronic infections which are now proven in everyone. These infections generally raise inflammation levels in the body, which tend to thicken the blood and impair oxygen delivery. This all contributes to our epidemic of degenerative diseases. Fortunately, I have located a safe and effective advanced form of oral silver called ACS (Advanced Cellular Silver) 200 that is at least 1,000 times more powerful than any other silver product available. This product helps me control the ubiquitous chronic infections proper testing reveals in all patients. ACS 200 silver is entirely safe so it can be taken in large doses for as long as needed, even for months, since chronic infections are not overcome easily. Most doctors ignore these ubiquitous chronic infections since they are so hard to eliminate with the outdated and ineffective antibiotics doctors rely on today.

Remember, I was born sick. The first couple of months, I barely survived. I ran high fevers. I was handicapped as a child, so it has been rather time-consuming, and expensive for me to achieve the high level of health I enjoy today. Once you have restored health, it is easier to maintain it, but I always have to be on an extensive supplement program. I also require lifetime hormone support including testosterone. We are clearly designed to reach 120 years of age. It's just that most of us never really knew that. Therefore, we spend our money on new television sets. We think we need a newer car and a bigger house. Most of us aren't aware that it takes money to achieve optimal health.

. . . .

Dr. Kondrot: Don't you think it's important to be tested for heavy metals, either by the urine challenge or some other method to identify what metals are elevated so you can then prescribe a specific detox treatment?

Dr. Gordon: Absolutely. In environmental medicine, you find many people who have had occupational exposures that they're not aware of. The test is always useful, but it's a little disappointing when you learn that the research at Harvard shows that there is no correlation between bone lead and levels found in the blood, urine, and hair. The point is you have two different categories of risk. One is people who might be working with heavy metals and not even be aware of it. For them, testing is useful without question because some are working and being exposed to higher-than-normal levels of toxins. The other category is everyone else, because we are all born toxic. It's important for people to know that you're not off the hook if your doctor looks at your hair test, blood, or provoked urine mineral test and says, "Nothing is coming out." That does not mean you do not need detoxing, but in fact, it usually suggests that you have some blocked detox pathways because all of us have toxins in us that are taking 20 to 30 years off our life spans.

. . . .

Dr. Kondrot: Please share with us some examples of patients you've treated over the years and how their health dramatically improved after undergoing a chelation or detox program.

Dr. Gordon: It's so rewarding. When I started in this field some 40 years ago, people were having major bypass surgery done left and right. Many people weren't surviving, so I was gratified when I could place all of my patients on my chelation protocol and tell them, "Don't go near the bypass surgeon. He is absolutely not needed no matter what your tests show." That was a strong position, but I had the data to show the harm surgery was doing and the safety of my administering 30 to 50 intravenous chelation treatments. I wish everyone could experience a series of IV EDTA infusions, but the original protocol that I developed for all chelating doctors took nearly three hours per session, so that caused many to delay getting chelated until they were in serious trouble

I was able to determine that for 98 percent of my patients, I could offer short IV chelation lasting 5 to 15 minutes instead, so patients can get back to work. Today, I often combine my newer, short chelation IV using calcium EDTA preferably followed with a five minute infusion of vitamins and minerals like magnesium called a Myer's Cocktail. That puts good things in and the chelation takes bad things out.

This simple 15-minute process can be helpful if given at first twice a week or so and then continued for a longer time, even if only done once or twice a month. I have been blessed to help my patients avoid fatal heart attacks now for many years. This is true even for patients who had been scheduled for immediate surgery as their tests indicated they were high risk.

I still cancel their surgery as long as they agree to stay on a lifetime of the special advanced oral chelation program I have developed called BCI. This program is based on my collaboration many years ago with Dr. Lester Morrison who was in charge of a $10 million research project at the Arteriosclerosis Research Institute at Loma Linda University. His oral cardiovascular support formula had been documented to reduce fatal heart attacks by 91 percent. When I added my chelation protocol to his program, it succeeded in preventing fatal heart attacks. I have been fortunate to not get phone calls saying, "Dr. Gordon's program didn't work, and my husband died," or "I lost two patients last week." I have not heard of any patient suffering from a fatal heart attack or stroke who has consistently followed my chelation protocol for many years. In subsequent years, I have continued to upgrade the formula with additional nutrients, for example, when the need for Essential Fatty Acids became firmly established.

Over my 56 years of practice, it has been very gratifying to be able to tell people, "Cancel that surgery because if you are alive when you get in my office, I am starting you on my program. Within two days of the oral chelation, you are protected." I explained that the standard tests for blocked arteries are misleading because, no matter how bad they look, the body almost always has tiny blood vessels their angiograms do not see. Pet scans are far more accurate to determine whether or not there is a part of your heart that is really screaming for blood. Generally, I found the PET shows no urgent need for any operation, but even if it does show an area with little blood flow, I still generally do not recommend surgery because I have been in practice now for 56 years and involved for 40 years with chelation. One of the most satisfying parts of my medical practice is being able to explain to patients that they don't need a bypass or stent. They do need help, but seldom do they ever require a stent or bypass surgery if they can adhere to my total program.

Part of what we're doing with oral chelation is keeping our patients' blood the thickness of water or wine and not let it become the thickness of ketchup. Thicker blood means increased tendency to make blood clots. Blood clots are the major trigger that leads to strokes and heart attacks. I can avoid those clots when I have my patients protected by the heparin-like action from natural substances called mucopolysaccarides. By keeping patients on my oral chelation program, which makes the blood much less thick and sticky, it also reduces the workload of the heart. Blood vessels are not stressed; oxygen carrying capacity is increased; all of which means I'm adding additional years to their lifespan. I take all my patients off

Coumadin or any other blood thinners as they are all very dangerous, and I can get the needed effect using my advanced special oral chelation program.

Other exciting points in my career are sometimes like detective stories. For example, I was able to help solve a problem with a lead smelting plant in Sacramento, California, where my nurse's husband worked. She had seen the successes we were having in my office with people coming from around the world. One day she said, "Do you mind if I check my husband? His fellow workers are often in the hospital for a month at a time, and they're always sick." I said, "By all means. Just bring a piece of hair in. We'll check it." It turned out to be off the scale with a high level of lead. That lab test put me in the middle of a legal issue because that level of lead poisoning meant there was a company in town that didn't know what it was doing. Before I did anything else, I tested two more workers, and they were loaded with lead. It turned out Kaiser Hospital had never diagnosed lead in any of those people who were frequently in the hospital for two and three weeks at a time until they got a little bit better and could go home.

Helping to uncover that critical situation was extremely gratifying. There are a lot of success stories. That's why I became medical director of what at the time was the largest mineral testing laboratory in the world. I kind of became a medical detective because with the hair and other mineral tests I could often find the solution. Sometimes it was not just elevated toxic metals; often there were also deficient levels of essential minerals like magnesium and zinc. We do not need all the excess calcium supplements people are taking because, over time, calcium makes the arteries harden. If you must take calcium, never do it without lots of magnesium.

I saved the life of a patient who actually had the highest level of cadmium I've ever seen. We were doing a special study for the Canadian government. The government was interested in finding out if Shell Oil was poisoning people as a result of taking the sour gas out of the sweet gas, and it turned out the answer was yes. In that study, this one hair test came back showing cadmium way off the scale. I managed to find that patient. She was in a big hospital. They were about to treat her for cancer. I said, "If you treat her, she'll be dead. She doesn't have cancer. She has cadmium poisoning." The result was that they listened to me. I have story after story. Remember, I've done several thousand cases. There's always that wild outlier. In one house, everybody living there had mercury poisoning. It was an amazing story. The grandmother liked to play with mercury, and she kept that shiny stuff in the kitchen drawer with the towels. The towels were poisoning all the dishes when they'd use a towel to wipe them.

. . . .

Dr. Kondrot: You've been actively involved over the years developing products for chelation, and you have a lot of your favorite products. What are some products people should be aware of and how should they take them?

Dr. Gordon: I want everybody to be aware that I have children who, when they are bathed in EDTA, absolutely love the bath for the first time and want to be bathed again and again. The parents tell me, "Wow. It's making a difference."

I use EDTA daily and in every form that I can, whether in the vein or in tablets. When I put it in tablets, I add additional things to it and call it my Essential Daily Defense. I add things like garlic and vitamin C. Essential Daily Defense is something anyone can safely take every day of their life. Sometimes people think they will be deprived of zinc and other things their body needs with chelation. I overcame that problem by putting my tablets into a package, so I always give everyone a powerful multiple-mineral supplement.

When I looked beyond that and realized how important the essential fatty acids were, I put them into a package. I not only had the tablets to put the good stuff in and the Essential Daily Defense to take the bad stuff out, but I added the essential oils. That became my Beyond Chelation Improved. It's now called Binding Cellular Impurities.

We were fortunate to have Gervasio Lamas of the Miami Heart Institute get government funding for the $31 million Trial to Assess Chelation Therapy (TACT). When he did the study, they had to publish it in the *Journal of the AMA* admitting that chelation is both safe and effective. There will be a second study.

As we look at the big picture, I realize there are many other toxins, so I developed what I call a power drink. My power drink, besides vitamin C, also includes organic greens with around 13 different varieties of cereal grass, vegetable and sea greens, things like spirulina, and cilantro which is a natural detoxifier. There are such good things in greens, and so many of us are deficient because we fail to eat them. My power drink also contains a special fiber that I developed. The fiber has in it beta sitosterol that helps take out fat-soluble poisons. Many of the poisons we've talked about today are going to be helped by chelation, but we have many other poisons that include dioxins and PCBs. There are so many others; the list is long. I also add a Peruvian root powder called MACA, and a product called Zeolite Enhanced to my Power Drink. Zeolite is an incredibly powerful detoxifier. It is even used to filter out radioactive compounds from water and soil. Zeolite has been around for many, many years, and we've been able to prepare it in a way that brings it to a unique level in treating health issues. Our zeolite product has been approved in over 40 countries. I really do want our Earth to go on, and everyone on the planet needs some oral detoxification every day of his or her life. Zeolite is one of the best detoxifiers.

Then we have exciting things to help hormone issues. For example, we now know that your bones are where your body stores the lead. If you're a woman, I will give you my herbal remedy from Thailand. It is Pueraria mirifica. Women will go through menopause more safely and experience less hypertension when they take this herb. In other words, when women's bones are melting away because they're going into menopause and they've lost their estrogen, that's when the doctor says, "I have to put you on a drug. Your blood pressure is high." The reason their blood pressure is high is because the lead stores are being released from their bones faster. Pueraria mirifica, as found in H.R.T. Plus, helps with a variety of menopausal symptoms like depression, headaches, and weak bones. Pueraria is also protective against breast cancers, and it helps a woman's bones stay strong. There is no depression; there is no insomnia, loss of memory, or Alzheimer's. It is an amazing herb.

Because of my worldwide travels and having had offices in Asia and Europe, I have learned about things that are not widely known in our country. I'm very optimistic that even though we've poisoned our planet, if people start to change their priorities, then they can do as I'm doing— having a healthy and happy life even starting at 80.

· ·

Dr. Kondrot: I'm curious about the EDTA in the bathtub. I think it's a novel and amazing approach. Can you tell us a little more about this?

Dr. Gordon: We've been adding EDTA to the bath water to help draw the toxins out of the skin, which is the largest organ of excretion, and our skin is loaded with metals. That's why the hair test is so useful. Toxins and metals can be concentrated as much as 20 times more in the hair. It became obvious that you could get a benefit from bathing in anything that can detoxify, so I have people bathe in zeolite powder one day, switch to Epsom salts the next day, and then I have a product called Beyond Bath with EDTA for another day.

. . . .

Dr. Kondrot: What would you say are the top three things you would like to see everyone who reads this chapter do for their health?

Dr. Gordon: If we can get more people on an oral formula based on my BCI (Binding Cellular Impurities), we can dramatically reduce the incidence of heart attack and strokes. This formula is a potent multivitamin and mineral formula packet containing ten capsules, including omega 3, primrose oil, and EDTA. Taken even just once a day by less ill patients, this formula can dramatically improve the health of our nation.

However, even if on BCI, we still need to take extra vitamin C, of which I take eight grams daily. I use BioEnRGy C, a hi-potency vitamin C that has been specially formulated with an internal delivery system so that it works almost like getting an infusion of vitamin C in the vein. It includes trimethylglycine, methyl sulfonyl methane, ribose, and essential sugars from Aloe vera.

I have determined that in order to capture and excrete as many toxins as possible, it is best to use a variety of chelators and detoxifiers, so I also recommend using zeolite. Zeolite has a magnetic affinity for toxic heavy metals like mercury, and it actually scavenges it more readily than EDTA.

My top three choices are BCI, BioEnRGy C, and ZeoGold Enhanced, products that provide some powerful armor that helps protect us while living on a poisoned planet.

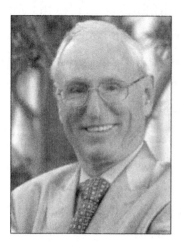

Garry F. Gordon, MD, DO, MD(H)
Gordon Research Institute
10915 Crestview Drive
Fountain Hills, AZ 85268
928-978-4424
Info@gordonresearch.com
www.gordonresearch.com

CHELATION AND ESTROGEN THERAPY: DOUBLE PROTECTION FOR WOMEN

Interview with
Marina Johnson, MD

Marina Johnson, M.D., FAC., a UCLA-USC trained physician, is a board certified endocrinologist and pharmacist with 30 years of clinical experience. She's published Outliving Your Ovaries: An Endocrinologist Reviews the Risks and Rewards of Treating Menopause with Hormone Replacement Therapy. *She's the medical director of the Institute of Endocrinology and Preventive Medicine in Dallas, Texas.*

Dr. Johnson practices integrative medicine, specializing in bioidentical hormone replacement for women and men, treatment of thyroid, adrenal and growth hormone disorders, cardiovascular prevention, and chelation therapy. She utilizes a holistic approach to determine the root cause of a patient's symptoms. While knowledgeable in pharmaceutical therapy, she believes in providing patients safe, effective natural therapies whenever possible. Dr. Johnson is passionate about patient education to empower patients to actively participate in their care.

1. **If a man's testosterone went to zero at age 50, he would insist that something be done to correct that problem. Why should it be any different for women?**

2. The common denominator in all degenerative disease is chronic inflammation.

3. One dental amalgam filling releases 3 to 17 micrograms per day, and this can exceed the FDA limit.

. . . .

Dr. Kondrot: Please tell us about your medical training.

Dr. Johnson: I'm an endocrinologist, a physician who specializes in hormones. I earned my undergraduate degree in pharmacy at the University of Houston. I then became Assistant Editor of the *American Hospital Formulary Service-Drug Information (AHFS-DI)*, a drug reference book published by the American Society of Hospital Pharmacists. *AHFS-DI* is a non-commercial book of monographs on every brand and generic drug that's available in the United States. My job was to research the medical literature and prepare comprehensive monographs on each drug. *AHFS-DI* has been officially adopted by the United States Public Health Service and the American College of Physicians as a recommended book for every internist's library. I enjoyed my work as an assistant editor because I love learning, but going to medical school gave me the opportunity to apply all this knowledge in a more useful manner.

I earned my medical degree from the University of California at Los Angeles and completed a three-year internal medicine residency at UCLA/St. Mary's Medical Center in Long Beach, California. Next I completed a two-year fellowship in endocrinology and metabolism at the University of Southern California in Los Angeles. After my fellowship, I worked at City of Hope Research Hospital in southern California for a couple of years. Then I decided to come home to Texas, and I've been in private practice ever since.

. . . .

Dr. Kondrot: What first made you interested in integrative medicine?

Dr. Johnson: When I first went into practice, I thought I knew everything. Then I realized that medical school only gives physicians the basic tools for evaluating patients. Becoming a skilled physician requires not only applying those tools but also carefully listening to the patient, ongoing study, and a commitment to lifelong learning.

One day about five years into my practice, I was referred a patient sent from her primary care physician. He told her, "I don't know what's wrong with you, but I'm sending you to Dr. Johnson. If she can't help you, you'll need to see a psychiatrist!" When I saw the patient, I knew she didn't have an endocrine problem, but I also knew she didn't have a psychiatric problem. That's when my practice took a major turn from traditional medicine. I was bound and determined to help this poor woman, and it started me on a quest to truly understand the body. Even then, I knew the body doesn't lie. Every sign and symptom means something. Signs and symptoms are your body's way of telling you what it needs. The body has an amazing capacity to heal itself. In most instances, when you correct the underlying root cause, the body heals, and the signs and symptoms resolve themselves.

. . . .

Dr. Kondrot: I understand you specialize in bioidentical hormones for women and men. What prompted you to focus on that?

Dr. Johnson: About ten years into my practice, I observed that women were being referred for diabetes or thyroid problems, but they were also suffering from menopausal symptoms no one was addressing. Because every woman goes through menopause, it's often not even considered a medical problem. Even today, women are often patted on the head and told, "Honey, you're getting older and you just need to go home and live with it." Well, I assure you if a man's testosterone went to zero at age 50, he would insist that something be done to correct that problem. Why should it be any different for women? I felt that women deserved to have the same consideration, so I started treating menopause as any other hormone deficiency.

It's been an incredible journey, and I've been blessed to participate in the transformation that occurs when a woman is made whole again. Today, about 70 percent of my practice consists of women of all ages. I see young women with premenstrual syndrome and other menstrual disorders, but most of my patients are women ages 40 to 60. Men can experience a decline in testosterone as they approach their 40s, and they comprise about 30 percent of my practice. For both men and women, I address thyroid, adrenal, and growth hormone disorders. Because heart disease is the number one killer of people over 50, I also focus on cardiovascular prevention.

. . . .

Dr. Kondrot: Why is heart disease so common in people over 50?

Dr. Johnson: As we age, there's an increase in degenerative diseases like heart disease and dementia. The common denominator in all degenerative disease is chronic inflammation. Inflammation is a normal process our immune system uses to repair our tissues after acute injuries and to protect us against infections. However, as we age, we acquire an increasing load of toxins that weakens our immune system leading to chronic inflammation. I first became aware of the importance of chronic inflammation in heart disease ten years ago by studying with Dr. Bradley Bale, an international expert in cardiovascular prevention. Dr. Bale has developed the Bale Doneen Method that identifies and treats the root cause of the cardiovascular disease to control the chronic inflammation. I found his method very useful in helping my patients with prevention of heart attacks and strokes.

. . . .

Dr. Kondrot: How did you become interested in chelation?

Dr. Johnson: Since I was already doing cardiovascular prevention, chelation was a logical development on my part to look for other ways of preventing heart disease. I had first heard about chelation 15 years ago, but, at the time, there were few scientific published studies supporting its use, so I was reluctant to use it. Then 12 years ago, the National Institutes of Health began a study called the Trial to Assess Chelation Therapy (TACT) to evaluate whether chelation had benefit in treating heart disease. TACT was set up as a randomized placebo-controlled trial that's considered to be the definitive way to conduct a scientific study. In 2013, the results of the TACT trial were published in the *Journal of the American Medical Association*. TACT studied the use of a drug called ethylenediamine tetra-acetic acid (EDTA) given as an intravenous (IV) infusion. The study included 1,700 patients with known heart disease who were followed for five years. All the patients received standard of care treatment for their heart disease like statins and blood pressure drugs. Half the group also received a weekly IV EDTA chelation for 30 weeks followed by ten monthly IV EDTA chelations. Those receiving EDTA also received either high-dose vitamins or placebo vitamins. The other half was given a placebo IV either with placebo vitamins or high-dose vitamins.

· ·

Dr. Kondrot: What were the findings in the TACT trial?

Dr. Johnson: I explain the results to my patients by using the statistical term NNT that stands for Number Needed to Treat. NNT is a way of explaining scientific findings in general terms that are easy for everyone to understand. The NNT for a therapy states how many people need to be treated over a five-year period to receive a benefit from that treatment.

For example, with a standard heart medicine like a statin, 25 to 30 patients need to be treated every day for five years to achieve one cardiac event reduction in a five-year period. When you look at the TACT trial, the NNT in diabetics treated with EDTA chelation and high-dose vitamins was only 5.5. In the diabetic subset that received EDTA chelation and no vitamins, the NNT was 7. In the entire group of diabetics and non-diabetics who were treated with EDTA chelation and high-dose vitamins, the NNT was 12. In the entire group of diabetics and non-diabetics treated with EDTA chelation and no vitamins, the NNT was 18. It appears that the reason that diabetics did so well with chelation is that chelation seems to be of most benefit to patients with microvascular heart disease. That's a hallmark of diabetic heart disease.

When you compare chelation with the drugs currently available, these results are phenomenal. It's important to emphasize that in any group of patients with heart disease, diabetics always have the worse outcome. Yet in the TACT trial, diabetics had the best outcome. Diabetics had a 39 percent reduction in heart disease and their deaths were reduced by 43 percent. Last but not least, there were no adverse events reported from EDTA chelation. So what's not to like about a therapy that's this effective and safe? In good conscience, how could I not offer this therapy to my patients? That's why I have now become certified and credentialed by two different organizations, ACAM and ICIM, to provide chelation.

· ·

Dr. Kondrot: How does a person know if he or she would benefit from

chelation?

Dr. Johnson: It's important for people to know that blood tests for toxic metals like lead or mercury are usually normal unless someone's had an accidental exposure. Because these metals are so harmful, the body deposits them in bone or other organs to reduce the immediate damage. That's why it's better to do a urine test called a Provocation Test for Toxic Metals. What amazes me is that almost every patient whom I've tested has come back with a significant burden of mercury, lead, and other toxic metals. We live in a toxic world. People often have no clue that they are loaded with toxic metals. The most common and harmful metals are lead and mercury.

. . . .

Dr. Kondrot: Where would people become exposed to these metals? Is that something people are exposed to in the workplace?

Dr. Johnson: Let's talk first about lead. It's true that certain occupations like electricians, plumbers, painters, and artists have increased exposure, but that's actually a small percentage of the people who have excessive lead. From Dr. Dorothy Merritt, a chelation expert in Houston, I learned that lead is much more pervasive. Let me give you some examples of where we get lead exposure.

1. Air from indoor dust exposure has a greater lead content than soil or paint chips.

2. Twenty percent of our daily exposure comes from "lead-free" brass fixtures that actually contain five to seven percent lead.

3. Lead is also found in some Ayurveda and foreign medicines and in cosmetics like lipsticks. While the amount of lead in lipsticks may not be huge, when you consider that girls start wearing lipstick at 12 and use it for the next 60 or more years, that daily exposure can add up.

4. Imported goods like red and yellow lead-glazed dishware, leaded crystal, and wine contain lead. Of 432 wines tested in the bottle, domestic wines ranged from 1 to 521 parts per billion, with an average

of 41. Imported wines ranged from 4 to 673 parts per billion with an average of 94. Did you know that a leaded crystal decanter leaches 2500-5500 mcg/l of lead in 24 hours? For comparison, the EPA limit for lead in drinking water is 50 parts per billion or 50 mcg/liter.

Dr. Kondrot: How are we exposed to mercury?

Dr. Johnson: Mercury is actually a common toxic metal that comes from dental amalgams, the so-called silver fillings that are actually 50 percent mercury. Mercury also comes from fish, coal-fired plants, and vaccines. The EPA says that a safe daily intake of mercury should not exceed 5.4 micrograms for a 120-pound woman and 7.5 micrograms for a 165-pound man. Did you know that one dental amalgam filling releases 3 to 17 micrograms per day? The fish containing the highest amount of mercury are the large fish like swordfish, shark, and king mackerel.

Dr. Kondrot: Is EDTA chelation related to detoxification?

Dr. Johnson: EDTA chelation is actually a type of detoxification because we're removing toxic metals that are very damaging to the body. All United States government agencies including the FDA, EPA, OSHA, and CDC agree there are no safe levels of lead and mercury. Both lead and mercury lead to atherosclerosis, high blood pressure, coronary heart disease, cardiomyopathy, strokes, and peripheral arterial disease. Traditional medicine currently provides no other therapy that addresses the removal of toxic metals.

Endocrinology involves the study of metabolism. Detoxification is also an important metabolic process of the body. We take in nutrients to repair cells and make new cells and, in the process, we generate waste products. There has to be an orderly mechanism for removing these waste products. The body itself is like a little machine that generates waste products. Removing these waste products and other toxins enables the body to perform more efficiently.

Dr. Kondrot: Tell me how you approach detoxification and which measures people can follow right now to improve their health.

Dr. Johnson: You need to consider the different factors that make a body healthy. Start by first putting in healthy food and supporting the natural processes the body has in place to keep itself clean and rid of toxins. Avoiding processed food and grains, especially genetically modified foods (GMO) is important. Eating a diet that's primarily organic fruits and vegetable and grass-fed organic meats reduces the number of toxins that are taken in on a daily basis. Foods like beets, radishes, artichokes, cabbage, broccoli, and chlorella help the liver to detoxify. Periodically, you can do a juice fast where you only take in fresh fruit and vegetable juices for three to seven days.

Having regular elimination is also required for detoxification because this is a major way the body removes toxins. A person should have at least two formed bowel movements a day. This can usually be achieved with a fiber-rich diet, probiotics, magnesium, and an adequate intake of water.

Water, the universal solvent, is essential for detoxification because the cells use water for the efficient removal of toxins. The average human adult body is 50 to 65 percent water. Your intake should be at least half your body weight in ounces of water. For a 130-pound woman, this would be 65 ounces or about eight glasses of water. The water should be pure, filtered water; at the very least reverse osmosis, but preferably filtered, alkaline water.

With my patients, I often use the following analogy. If someone told you, "I'm giving you this nice home, but it's the only one you'll ever have." When it came time to repair that home, would you go to the junkyard and repair it with discarded lumber or poor quality materials? Of course not, you would go to the store and select the finest building materials because that house has to last for the rest of your life. Remember that everything you put in your body becomes you. Do you want to build new brain cells with fake fat from McDonald's? Would you let the floors of your house pile up with garbage?

Sweating provides another route for eliminating toxins. This can be achieved through regular exercise or saunas. My favorite sauna is the far infrared sauna. Sleep enables your body to rest and repair, and adults need seven to eight hours of sleep. The liver, an important organ for detoxification, is most active between 1:00

and 3:00 a.m. Herbs like dandelion root, burdock, and milk thistle are protective of the liver.

Reduce stress by eliminating toxic emotions like anger and lack of forgiveness. Adopt the daily habit of showing gratitude. People who exhibit gratitude as a permanent trait rather than a temporary state of mind have healthier immune systems and cope better with stress. A 1995 study in the *American Journal of Cardiology* showed that appreciation and positive emotions are linked with improvements in heart rate variability that can be beneficial in the treatment of hypertension and in reducing the likelihood of sudden death in patients with congestive heart failure and heart disease.

. . . .

Dr. Kondrot: Since you're a hormone specialist, I know you treat menopause with natural bioidentical hormones. Does estrogen have a role in protecting against heart disease?

Dr. Johnson: Absolutely! Estrogen is why premenopausal women always have lower heart disease rates than men of the same age. Postmenopausal women who use estrogen have 32 percent less heart disease and improve their mortality by 39 percent. Estrogen has at least eight ways in which it protects a woman's cardiovascular system: it increases HDL, the good cholesterol, and reduces LDL, the bad cholesterol; it improves blood pressure; it reduces excess clotting in the blood; it dilates arteries to improve blood flow; it's anti-inflammatory; it reduces insulin resistance; it's a natural calcium channel blocker; and it prevents plaque formation.

People often think of heart disease as a man's disease but according to American Heart Association statistics, more women died last year of heart attacks than men. Women are most fearful of breast cancer, but from 2007 NIH statistics, 450,000 women died of heart disease and stroke compared to 48,000 women who died of breast cancer.

Women with heart disease are often misdiagnosed because their presenting symptoms are atypical. Instead of having classic chest pain like men, women may exhibit shortness of breath or unusual fatigue. When women undergo angiograms, they are often normal, which further obscures their diagnosis. A 2005 study in the *Journal of the American Medical Association* showed that women admitted with an acute heart attack had a two-fold increase in "normal" coronary arteries compared to men. This condition has been termed Microvascular Coronary Dysfunction because it involves disease in the capillaries, the microcirculation. The microcirculation delivers oxygen and nutrients to all the cells and is 76 percent of the entire circulatory system. Men are more likely to have obstructive coronary disease.

. . . .

Dr. Kondrot: Is there any connection between estrogen and EDTA chelation?

Dr. Johnson: There is a connection in that EDTA and estrogen are both protective of the heart. However, while EDTA is a drug, as we just discussed, estrogen is an essential component of a woman's body. When estrogen drops at menopause, lead that's stored in bone is released and can worsen heart disease. It makes a lot of sense to give both because chelation and estrogen are additive therapies that can be synergistic. Recall that the TACT trial showed the most dramatic benefits in patients with diabetes. Heart disease in diabetics is also a disease of the microcirculation. Because EDTA chelation was so beneficial in treating the microvascular disease of diabetics, it should prove to be an especially useful therapy in women.

The TACT trial showed great benefit for EDTA chelation in reducing heart disease measured by fewer heart attacks, fewer hospitalizations, and reduced mortality. Taking estrogen reduces heart disease in postmenopausal women by 32 percent. Because women's heart disease is primarily microvascular, women should have further benefit by adding chelation to their estrogen therapy.

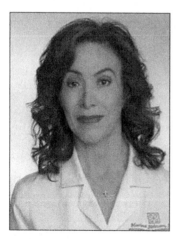

Marina Johnson, M.D., FACE,
Medical Director
Institute of Endocrinology and Preventive
Medicine
Dallas, TX 75206
www.drmarinajohnson.com

THERE ARE MANY WAYS TO DETOXIFY AND RESTORE VISION

Interview with
Edward Kondrot, MD, MD(H), CCH, DHt, FCSO

Dr. Kondrot is the world's leading homeopathic ophthalmologist who devotes his practice to traditional and alternative therapies for the treatment of eye disease. He is president of the Arizona Homeopathic and Integrative Medical Association (AHIMA) and he is the clinic director of the American Homeopathic Medical College. Dr. Kondrot's two best-selling books, Healing the Eye the Natural Way *and* Microcurrent Stimulation: Miracle Eye Cure, *are solid introductions into his philosophy and practice. His latest book,* 10 Essentials to Save Your Sight, *has received rave reviews. He is the host of the weekly radio show* Healthy Vision *broadcast on KFNX Talk Radio.*

Healing the Eye and Wellness Center provides proven and effective alternative treatments for eye conditions, including macular degeneration, cataracts, and glaucoma. Dr. Kondrot's seminars and three-day restore vision program have become the standard in alternative therapies for eye disease.

In October 2014, Dr. Kondrot received the Academy of Comprehensive Integrative Medicine's Lifetime Achievement Award for work in alternative therapies in the treatment of eye disease.

1. I tell patients, "You could be dying of lead and mercury poisoning, and if you check your urine and blood, it's going to be normal." The lead and mercury don't stick around in your urine and blood. They go into your bones, muscles, fat, brain, and eyes.

2. I felt this was a second reason to do chelation – to remove the toxic heavy metals that had an adverse effect on the retinal tissue, the lens, and the health of the eye.

3. Through testing, we can get a list of hundreds of different products that have adversely affected the patient. What do we do with those products? We imprint them into a homeopathic remedy.

. . . .

Dr. Courtney: Take us through your medical training and the journey that brought you to the point where you are today.

Dr. Kondrot: My career started as a traditional medical doctor. I went to school at Hahnemann Medical College in Philadelphia, and I fell in love with ophthalmology. I found that I had a special gift, a special surgical skill. When I finished my ophthalmology residency, I felt there wasn't an eye that I could not put back together. I was young and single at the time, and I joined the trauma service at Allegheny General Hospital. They had one of the largest trauma hospitals in the area. I was on call, and I would go in at night to take care of people who had been in automobile accidents and other serious traumatic cases. I felt I could restore any eye. Eventually my practice evolved into a more traditional ophthalmology practice doing cataract surgery, corneal transplants, and glaucoma surgery.

I was very good at what I did, but my practice began to change. After a while, I'd see patients who I thought I had helped, and they would come back with some type of chronic problem, or the surgical correction did not hold. The glaucoma returned. The cataract led to macular degeneration. I began to question whether there might be a better method.

Right around this time, I got a phone call from my uncle, a dairy farmer in Pennsylvania. He was told that he had triple-vessel vascular disease, and he needed open-heart surgery at the very same hospital where I was on staff. The operation would cost over $100,000, and he didn't have any insurance.

He asked me if I had ever heard of chelation. Of course, the only time I heard of chelation in my medical training was in a very disparaging manner—calling it quackery and a waste of the patient's money. I was kind to my uncle and said, "I really haven't heard anything good about it, but I can understand your situation. Why don't you try the chelation to see if it can help you? I don't think it's going to hurt you." He did. He underwent a series of chelation treatments, and his chest pain resolved. He was able to return to work on the dairy farm without any problems, and he was doing very well.

I became curious about chelation. I was talking to one of my colleagues with whom I did my ophthalmology residence, Dr. Harold Behar, who practices in Philadelphia. From what I remembered about Harold, he was very conservative. During our conversation, I found out he was doing chelation for macular degeneration. I said, "Harold, why in the world are you doing chelation? I thought it was just for heart disease. It's even questionable for that." He said, "I'm getting good results. It's turning macular degeneration patients around."

After that, I decided to investigate this. I joined ACAM, the American College for Advancement in Medicine, and took their chelation certification. I began doing chelation therapy in my practice. Much to my surprise, just about every eye patient I treated had some improvement in his or her vision. The chelation didn't cure the macular degeneration, but it was a method I could use to help these folks when I didn't have anything else to offer them, aside from vitamins and monitoring their vision. Chelation therapy became an important part of my practice.

Chelation therapy has a double meaning behind it. There is the chelation that the ACAM doctors teach. That technique was designed for cardiovascular benefit, for improving blood flow to various areas, and it can do all that. Then, of course, there's chelation for removing metals.

. . . .

Dr. Courtney: When did you begin to see the metals themselves as the

problem and that detoxification was needed? From your clinical viewpoint, would you say the metals became more important than the blood flow?

Dr. Kondrot: Before I answer that, the story gets even more interesting. My uncle, who had responded well with chelation, was now working back on the dairy farm, and he didn't continue with his maintenance chelation. The doctor who was treating him wanted him to come back every month for maintenance, but my uncle felt great and didn't return.

His chest pain came back. He was unable to work, but now he had insurance, so he decided to take care of the problem surgically. Interestingly, his chest pain persisted. The doctors told him, "There's really no reason for the chest pain. All your vessels are open. It's psychological." He went back and had another series of chelation treatment and they took care of his chest pain. He was very upset because he felt that the open-heart surgery did absolutely nothing for him. It was the chelation that had helped. This was another bit of information that prompted me to explore chelation in a little more detail.

To answer your question about the heavy metals, as I began to look more deeply into the cause of macular degeneration, I began ordering six-hour urine challenge tests on my patients because I feel this is the only way to accurately measure heavy metals. I tell patients, "You could be dying of lead and mercury poisoning, and if you check your urine and blood, it's going to be normal." The lead and mercury don't stick around in your urine and blood. They go into your bones, muscles, fat, brain, and eyes. You need to take a chelating agent to make those toxic metals soluble, then they can be measured in your excreted urine. When I began doing six-hour challenge tests, I discovered that the vast majority of patients I was seeing with serious eye problems, like macular degeneration, cataracts, and glaucoma, had heavy metal loads that were off the chart. I felt this was a second reason to do chelation, not only to improve the blood flow to the eye and the vascular flow but also to remove the toxic heavy metals that had an adverse effect on the retinal tissue, the lens, and the health of the eye.

. . . .

Dr. Courtney: How did you see your patients respond as you began to focus on removing heavy metals?

Dr. Kondrot: It was frustrating for me because patients typically look at chelation therapy as a quick fix where, with one or two IV chelation treatments, all their heavy metals will be gone. After a series of 10 or 20 treatments, maybe we would see a slight reduction in the lead and mercury. That was kind of frustrating, not only for patients but also for me, so I began to look at other methods for removing these heavy metals.

Right around the time I was introduced to chelation, I was also introduced to microcurrent. I heard about microcurrent when I read that Sam Snead, the famous golfer, had a reversal of his macular degeneration using microcurrent. This was in the late '90s, and I began incorporating microcurrent into my practice. Microcurrent is a way to improve blood flow and stimulate cellular activity. Interestingly, it's also a way to help detoxification. It can help mobilize heavy metals. It can support the kidney, liver, and lymphatic system during any type of chelation process. Soon I made it part of my protocol with all the patients I was treating who had heavy metal poisoning and chronic eye disease to have some type of detoxification program using microcurrent in conjunction with chelation therapy.

The other thing I began to look at were other methods of delivering the EDTA. I was trained that IV therapy was the only way to remove heavy metals. Unfortunately, not everyone is willing to make the financial and time investment to have a series of 20 or 40 IV chelation therapies. I began to look at rectal chelation where we insert a suppository of EDTA, and it's absorbed into the rectal mucosa. It goes into the bloodstream. That has been shown to be effective. I was also looking at oral methods of chelation. I felt very strongly that all of my patients who had a serious eye problem needed to, first of all, identify what metals were elevated and then begin to do some type of chelation program in conjunction with microcurrent.

Around this time, I began using light therapy as a means of detoxification. That may seem strange to many people. How can light possibly help eliminate toxins in the body? There's an organization called the College of Syntonics that has, for the past 75 years, been using different wavelengths of light to help the eye regenerate and to detoxify the eye.

In our vascular system, we have an element called hemoglobin, a molecule that is almost identical in structure to chlorophyll. We all know that chlorophyll is the component of a plant that absorbs ultraviolet light and converts it to energy for the plant. In our vascular system, we have hemoglobin molecules that have the ability to absorb light and transform this light into energy into the vascular system to help improve oxygenation, energy, and detoxification.

Light therapy became an important part of my detoxification program. I am using some type of chelation therapy, microcurrent, and light therapy as detoxification methods. I feel that all of those modalities, when combined, have a synergistic effect and help patients get the best possible result.

. . . .

Dr. Courtney: You said the word "synergy," the right word here. All those modalities work on a patient's particular medical problem, whether it's only eye-related or there are other problems. The results must be exponentially better than any one of those methods when used alone.

Dr. Kondrot: I looked at a group of 150 patients over a two-year period, and I carefully studied all the data. I'm pleased to say that my research article was accepted for publication in the *Journal of Alternative Therapies in Health and Medicine.* Below is a summary of my research:

> The purpose of the research was to demonstrate the effectiveness of alternative modalities in improving vision in chronic eye conditions even when administered over a short-term period. One hundred fifty-two patients with 1 or more of 11 types of eye disease attended one three-day session I conducted at my Healing the Eye and Wellness Center near Tampa, Florida, over a two-year period (January 2011 – December 2012). The number of participants in each session ranged from 5 to 15 with 13 as the average. All participants remained in the study for the duration of the program.

> These 11 ocular conditions are ordinarily considered incurable by any method except surgery and, even with surgery, the outcomes can be variable and/or transient. Seventy-eight percent of the patients had either Age-Related Macular Degeneration or Glaucoma, which together are the leading cause of blindness in

persons over 65 years of age. Detailed medical, dietary, and lifestyle histories were taken at the beginning of the three days. The purpose of the sessions was to improve vision using alternative treatments of IV Nutrition, Oxidative Therapy, Microcurrent Stimulation, and Syntonic Light Therapy. Each participant received each modality in the protocol. Following the administration of the protocol, significant improvement in Acuity, Contrast, and Visual Field resulted in the majority of participants. None of the interventions was toxic or painful, and all likely contributed to an improved overall health status of the participants. Long-term follow-up studies are now in process.

I want to mention another technique I'm using. I learned this from Dr. Lee Cowden who developed a program that uses biofeedback. I'm seeing more and more patients where it's almost impossible to test them for harmful toxins that they have been exposed to, whether it's electromagnetic energy, pesticides, or various other environmental toxins. I think heavy metals are a big component, but we need to look at these other parameters. When it's impossible to do a laboratory test, how can you evaluate a person who has toxic symptoms?

There's a method called ZYTO biofeedback. To use this to assess toxins, we run 5,000-plus different frequencies of toxic parameters or toxic elements, and we see how the person responds. It's similar to kinesiology. If there is a negative resonance, the person will become weak, and that indicates that they are adversely affected by the substance being tested. If there's no effect, there will be no change in the energy of the person, and that means the person is not adversely affected by that substance. This does it very quickly through a hand-held cradle, a biofeedback device. The patient sits passively, and we test over 5,000 different compounds for each patient. Typically, we get a list of hundreds of different products that have adversely affected the patient. The question is what do we do with those products? We imprint this into a homeopathic remedy.

Homeopathy has always been a big part of my practice. I believe the body has the ability to heal, and homeopathy is based on the Law of Similars where a substance that causes a disease or problem can be used to treat that situation in a very dilute solution or low dose. We imprint the toxins the patient has been exposed to in a very low dose homeopathic solution. We don't have the patient drink or take this as a medication. We do laser detoxification with it. We shine a laser light through the solution, and then that light is aimed toward the person's skin. Then the homeopathic energy of detoxification acts as a catalyst to release the toxins and help the patient heal. I'm doing this on patients who are extremely toxic and on patients who just don't respond to the typical methods of microcurrent and intravenous, oral, or rectal chelation.

Dr. Courtney: What do you call that process?

Dr. Kondrot: It's called laser detoxification. Dr. Lee Cowden describes this method in some detail in his interview in this book. This is not something new. I first heard Dr. Cowden speak of this at a meeting in Arizona close to ten years ago. He has now developed the software protocols to make it much easier for a physician to begin to incorporate it into his or her practice.

Dr. Courtney: You're always open to newer therapies and are a great resource for us to discover what has really worked and proven effective. You've been helpful to my own development. Every time you write a new book, you emphasize the most current therapies in use, so other doctors and the public can know about them.

Dr. Kondrot: There's another technique I'm using that I think you'll find very fascinating. I believe that many patients have emotional blockages. Recent research shows that emotions somehow cause interference in the energy field of the human body. In some cases, no matter what physical therapies we institute, like removing the heavy metals or putting patients on the right vitamins and nutrients, the body just does not heal. By identifying these energy blockages and identifying and treating the associated emotions, we can have a dramatic improvement.

I think this is one of the mechanisms of homeopathy. It always fascinates me how one homeopathic remedy can make such a profound change in an individual. For example, I developed severe adult onset asthma about 20 years ago and almost died twice. I tried all the conventional medical treatments, my inhaler and theodore. I still was having asthmatic attacks. I also changed my diet, increased my hydration, did meditation and everything I could to try to lick this problem. One single homeopathic remedy cured me of my asthma, and it amazed me how a substance that was dilute beyond any physical measurement could do this. I think it did this by somehow changing my energetic field, and then my physical problem resolved.

I've been working with a very interesting doctor, Dr. Charles Crosby, who developed a scalar device. It helps locate energy blockages and treats them. This is something I'm beginning to use in my practice. I like to call it the emotional detox of the person.

. . . .

Dr. Courtney: What important information do you feel the public should know about heavy metals, metal or non-metal toxic substances, and detoxification in general?

Dr. Kondrot: The most important step individuals can take is to look closely at their diet. That is one of the greatest contributing factors to poor health in the United States. You really have to shift your diet toward organic, raw, living foods that have the natural ability to detoxify, and avoid genetically modified (GMO) food. You have to avoid processed food and high fructose corn syrup. Second, you have to increase your water intake. Water is one of the best ways of detoxifying your body. Most people walk around in a dehydrated state.

You also have to find a good, pure source of water. Drinking tap water is not the best way to go. Most people now understand that water in plastic bottles has harmful phthalates and benzene derivatives. I like the reverse osmosis machines. You can put them underneath your kitchen sink, and they provide a good, pure source of water.

The third step that people can take is to balance the autonomic nervous system and reduce stress to get rid of the emotional elements that are causing a toxic reaction in our bodies and in our lives. Taking care of the emotional body is one of the most important keys to maintaining or regaining health.

Once these three things are done, look at heavy metal poisoning. Contact a well-trained integrative doctor and get tested for heavy metals. Begin some type of chelation program to remove heavy metals if you have them. These are very important steps that everyone needs to take to help regain their health.

. . . .

Dr. Courtney: You enrich me every time we meet. You're helping the people who read this book appreciate the fact that there are new techniques coming into our practices to help clear out toxic agents, and, by doing this, they can regain their health.

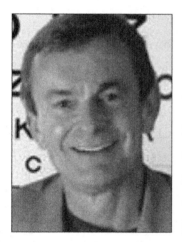

Edward Kondrot, MD, MD(H), CCH, DHt, FCSO
Director of the Florida Healing the Eye and Wellness Center
2666 Swamp Cabbage Court
Fort Myers, FL 33901
800-430-9328
www.HealingTheEye.com
info@HealingTheEye.com

DETOXIFY YOURSELF AND YOUR ENVIRONMENT FOR OPTIMAL HEALTH

Interview with
Jeffrey J. Kotulski, DO

Having studied Family Medicine, Jeffrey J. Kotulski, DO has been trained to provide comprehensive medical care for families and individuals suffering from all types of illnesses, disorders, conditions, and diseases. As a family doctor, Dr. Kotulski is usually the first point of contact for patients when they seek general medical care and can refer patients to specialists when necessary.

Member: American Osteopathic Association, American Academy of Osteopathy, American College of Osteopathic Family Physicians, American Academy of Anti-Aging Medicine, Cranial Academy, American Holistic Medical Association, Minnesota Osteopathic Medical Society, International Society of Orthomolecular Medicine, Institute of Functional Medicine

1. **Detoxification to me is both a macroscopic and microscopic event.**

2. **In one case, it took almost a year, but the child said, "I love you" to the mother.**

3. If somebody has an active cancer that's metastasized and is well advanced, we'll stress a ketogenic diet.

. . . .

Dr. Kondrot: **Dr. Kotulski, please tell us about your medical training and how you became interested in chelation and detoxification methods.**

Dr. Kotulski: My medical training started at the Chicago College of Osteopathic Medicine in 1987. Originally, my intention was to go into an allopathic training model, but after sitting in classes with a friend of mine who was attending a medical school in Chicago, I realized I was more interested in healthcare instead of sick care.

While waiting to enter osteopathic school, I received a master's degree in exercise physiology and cardiovascular health. I worked with populations who were sick and didn't necessarily respond to conventional medicine, so I saw firsthand that diet and exercise played a critical role in healing.

During my undergraduate training, I developed a bone marrow disorder. I had a very low white count as well as a low platelet count. I was given a treatment plan by a hematologist, but I sought out some orthomolecular physicians and was then put on a forever path of enhancing the innate healing potential within.

Since then, I have remained true to that notion. Even in osteopathic school, I questioned many things and often asked why we do things. It was frustrating when the reason given was that this is the way we've been doing it.

I chanced upon chelation after medical school, as most chelation therapists do. I studied it through various organizations—ACAM, the American Academy of Environmental Medicine, and the Institute for Functional Medicine. These influences have shaped my current practice toward orthomolecular medicine. Editor's Note: Orthomolecular medicine describes the practice of preventing and treating disease by providing the body with optimal amounts of substances which are natural to the body.

. . . .

Dr. Kondrot: One interesting thing is your strong farming background.

You know firsthand how food is raised. How do you relate that to your medical practice?

Dr. Kotulski: Farming—the concepts of farming and all it entails—has always intrigued me because that's the way humans can realize optimal health. I grew up in a suburb of Chicago, and my folks had been raised on dairy farms. I spent quite a few summers on the farm when I was young. It's very apparent when you're raising animals that you have to take care of many facets of the food chain, not just the food. You pay attention to the soil and to the micronutrients that are fed to the animals. When you looked at the animal in total, you came to really appreciate how vital appropriate food is for livestock. The contrast between this and what we do for ourselves struck me as peculiar from the beginning. We're willing to put all kinds of processed chemicals in our food and livestock without any knowledge of how those chemicals impact our bodies.

A simple example is what we've done to our livestock, in particular the dairy herds. We took a lifespan of 12 years of productivity on the dairy farm and reduced it to five years. I see parallels with humans because we now have chronic debilitating disease much earlier in our lives compared to the past. That's because of the altered food we now consume.

. . . .

Dr. Kondrot: Please share with us what advice you give to your patients who have a toxic load and may be suffering from chronic illnesses.

Dr. Kotulski: Detoxification in all its facets is critical for long-term survival, not just for us but also for the human species. Detoxification isn't just taking care of the liver or kidney or making sure we're perspiring. It's really taking care of our environment in total and making sure we're getting food, air, and water of a quality that's going to support us in continually cleansing ourselves.

Detoxification to me is both a macroscopic and microscopic event. For those who are in the depths of despair with chronic illness, detoxification becomes more microscopic, and we have to take care of the many facets of the liver's capacity to enhance detoxification. We sometimes have to go in depth, do DNA analysis, or do specific enzyme testing to figure out which pathways are not working properly.

The detoxification then becomes a matter of making choices regarding anything that interacts with us—the air we breathe, the food we eat, and the very thoughts we have. Emotions can make us toxic. We have to understand detoxification in a holistic sense. Once we do that, the healing starts. When we see an individual who is not optimally well, we look at not just the spiritual but also the energetics of what has comprised their life thus far. We can go back generations and find out that there's been a level of toxicity that has prevailed in their family. Now, in the present generation, it has become a significant toxic burden. If that's the case, we're going to have to work on this individual with a much different approach than just offering healing foods, sauna, and things like that. We're going to have to explore their mindset and look at their health in a generational perspective.

When we do that, we start to un-layer the issues. It is comparable to peeling the skin of an onion because there are often a lot of tears shed. In this process, the body goes through various pains. When the body comes to a point of balance again, there's sometimes an unsettling or reverberation that happens before we get in harmony again with the environment and with our own unique spirit.

Then we dig a little deeper. We become concerned with the flora within and with the microbiome. We start to get rid of toxins at the gut level. Sometimes they're pervasive. We have to get rid of infections throughout the body. Then we start to really hone in, get the liver pathways working well, get the kidney functioning optimally, and get the body moving. Once we start to do that, we get a purging of many toxins.

This is how we start to redirect the person from the path of destruction all the way over to a healing path. It's significant for individuals because now they have to adjust to a life that has potential to heal as opposed to a life that was breaking down. There is no scripted program for doing this. This is frustrating for mainstream medicine. When I teach residents, they ask, "What's your algorithm? What's your process? What do you do?" It's not a formula but a mindset you need to have that needs to be intertwined with the co-learner, the client who sits across from you. Everyone is different, but there are basic things we do. We introduce people to healthy foods, sauna, and gentle exercises. The most important thing we do is create—at least within our clinic—an environment where anxiety, agitation, irritation, and barriers are reduced or removed, so individuals can see themselves in a different light. They're not seeing a bleak or hopeless future. When it's all said and done, people end up with hope, and they move forward.

When individuals come into the clinic, sometimes we do an elaborate workup to determine their specific toxicity issues. Sometimes we just listen to them and find out that there is layer upon layer of toxicity. As a professional working with the client, I have to decide where we're going to intervene. I try to make a decision to intervene where there can be an impact. I'll often start with an elimination diet. Then we pre-tox—we open the pathways of elimination so the body can remove the toxins in a healthier manner.

. . . .

Dr. Kondrot: Please give an example of two patients where the approach has been different, perhaps for the same problems?

Dr. Kotulski: Let's go to the two ends of the spectrum of life. We'll take a child who has autism-like qualities in their behavior, and we'll contrast that to an elderly person.

In the example with the child, you have an individual who is basically locked in. They're not aware of their social setting. They don't communicate with their parents. There's no interaction with siblings. We look at that individual and make some general assessments. With regard to their diet, we try to figure out if they are addicted to certain foods. Are they showing signs of obvious allergic responses to foods? Then we look for history, and we glean that from the parents. What exposures did the mom have? What was going on when the child was in the womb?

We try to figure out if there's been any excessive exposure to heavy metals or plasticizers, which I call gender benders. They're things that cause endocrine disruption. It can give a young boy female characteristics to the extent that his hormone panel will be off, or vice versa, a female with high testosterone levels. Next, we get the individual eliminating very well regarding bowel movements and making sure they're hydrated. Then we look for any toxins. We may treat somebody for Lyme disease, heavy metal exposure, or other occult infections.

Then we enhance certain antioxidants in the body. We really try to enhance glutathione and R-lipoic acid. We add colon binders like calcium-d-glucarate.

Once that process is in place, we can be very specific with chelation if necessary. Then we work on oxidative stress in total. We may use hyperbaric oxygen therapy. We'll do other nutritional interventions and put the child on an elimination diet. Over time, there's going to be a change. The child who was basically locked in is now starting to interact with family. They may vocalize.

We had one example where it took almost a year, but the child said, "I love you" to the mother. The mother was so overwhelmed with her emotions. They were 50 miles or so from the clinic, and she made the husband turn around and come back. She was so ecstatic. The staff met them at the door upon their return and said, "So-and-so is back in the clinic." I thought, "Oh, boy. Something happened," in a not-so-positive way. She was crying. She told me the story, and then I was crying. You get those kinds of responses, but it's a process. It's not overnight.

From there, you can build upon that child's innate healing potential and get the child in school, back into mainstream education. There are many beautiful examples of children with developmental disorders or autism or who are on the spectrum who have had dramatic changes.

With an adult, it's sometimes not as impactful. Nonetheless, it can be quite enhancing to their vitality, enough so that they don't end up in a nursing home. I had a client in her 80s who broke her arm. She had done painting with her dad when she was a little girl, and her dad used paint containing lead. The lady became acutely psychotic after the break. It was quite clear there were acute changes with her mentation. Her serum lead level was elevated. We didn't even have to do a provocative test. She also developed atrial fibrillation. The magnesium in her body was displaced because of the lead. Her treatment plan consisted of taking care of the fracture, chelation for the lead, and IV magnesium to restore normal heart rhythm.

We do all the things that are safe, like an echocardiogram to make sure she's not developing a clot. She was placed on nattokinase, magnesium, D-ribose, CoQ10, and fish oil. We got rid of the lead, and she was able to stay home and recover rather than go to the nursing home and convalesce there. That's a case that illustrates how cost-effective we can be when we look at the person in total and we're aware of their history of toxic exposure.

Those are two cases at either end of the spectrum of life. Each was rather dramatic in the outcome and the way we were able to change the course of their current and future health.

. . . .

Dr. Kondrot: what is the biggest toxic threat that you see in your practice?

Dr. Kotulski: Right now, without a doubt, it's toxic food. I think simple things are making a major disturbance. We have evolved as a species to handle toxins, but we haven't figured out what to do with stuff like high-fructose corn syrup. High-fructose corn syrup is really an amped up sugar molecule, and the body does not process it the same way as it does a glucose molecule. It causes a significant amount of inflammation, and it causes insulin dysregulation at a much higher level. Because of that, we end up with distortion in the metabolic pathways. This leads not only to an epidemic of obesity, but it has also been linked to many of our chronic debilitating illnesses, such as osteoarthritis, gall bladder disease, cancer, heart disease, stroke, and Alzheimer's. We have a litany of conditions where we can say, "We have a pathway, and we have a potential culprit in high-fructose corn syrup." There are some other variables that are mixed into this, but by and large, it's high-fructose corn syrup. I think Dr. Robert Lustig in his books and lectures has illustrated this very eloquently to show that high-fructose corn syrup is responsible for the childhood obesity epidemic.

. . . .

Dr. Kondrot: Please continue commenting on how food contributes to our toxic society.

Dr. Kotulski: A lot of global research is being done on genetically modified food. In the United States, we're a little more biased with the information that gets out to the public. If you can open the mind a little bit and appreciate the international research, we're seeing strong links to cancer and obesity in GMO food. When you see the cancer incidence approaching one in two here in the United States, there's something going on. We can put our heads in the sand and continue to ignore what's going on, but there are some major disruptions in metabolism. There are endocrine disruptions because of the genetically modified food in an indirect way because now we have pesticides and insecticides that are used quite differently. So many studies show that we have an incredible amount of endocrine disruption.

With the infertility that's being bred into the population, we're going to have an unfortunate outcome of zero population growth. Eventually, our species is going to be forever altered. We've had a dramatic change in our fertility rates, at least here locally in southern Minnesota. It's quite alarming.

Some studies show that perhaps one in 25 females was infertile back in the early '90s. It's approaching one in four now. That's a change that is reminiscent of the Pottenger cat study. Dr. Francis Pottenger worked with a feline model looking at food that was corrupted or processed. After four generations, the cats fed the poorer diet were no longer able to breed. If you extrapolate that data to the human model, we're in the third generation right now. By the fourth generation, we become totally infertile. To me, that's an incredible change that's taking place.

We had zero population growth for Caucasians in the United States this last year, and nobody is alarmed by that. That's never happened before in the United States. We've had a very low teenage pregnancy rate, but the STD (Sexually Transmitted Disease) rate was actually very high, so it's not a matter of abstinence. It's a matter of infertility. We have a bigger problem than just obesity. We have a lot of endocrine disruption going on.

I'll mention this again. I call them gender benders—the toxins that can actually transform a little boy into a little girl and vice versa. The University of Chicago opened a transgender clinic in March of 2013 to deal with such issues. Nobody is getting overly excited about that. When I present that to doctors, most of them aren't even aware that the clinic was opened.

. . . .

Dr. Kondrot: What advice do you give to patients or readers about what they can do right now to improve their health and reduce their toxic load?

Dr. Kotulski: Jokingly, I say you can live in a glass bubble. The reality is that we are engulfed in toxins. They're within us and surrounding us. What you can do is make choices. You can make choices with the air you breathe, the food you consume, and the water you drink. If you're making choices that are healthier within those three parameters, you support your own internal detoxification processes.

If we're going to help the issue globally or in the local community, we're going to have to speak up and do something different with our wastewater and our food production. We're going to have to do something different with air quality. We're going to have to empower individuals and get people excited. We need to light a torch because we need a policy change and a social movement. We'll need to make market changes and shift what we do with our money because right now we value sickness. We have to start to value health and bring this awareness to the national and international level.

Patients can do many things. I had a patient who had advanced stage colon cancer. She wasn't given too many options with the traditional medical model. She went through our program, and she's thriving right now. She was aware that perhaps it was the food, the advanced glycation end products, and some of these other things that can sit in the colon, fester, and cause changes in the colon that caused her problem. Now she's opening a food co-op. That's inspiring. This individual was educated about diet through her therapy. She got excited and realized food was going to be her ticket to health. A guiding principle all of us who practice ortho-molecular or functional medicine have is "Let food be thy medicine."

That's what we do best at our clinic and what makes us a unique. When patients come to the office, right away they're met with food. Back where the health practitioners see patients, there's healthy food. There's a kitchen upstairs to teach them how to cook. We have a nutritionist who meets with them on their visits. All of our staff are trained in various forms of food, healing, and nurturing. If there's a question regarding food, our staff can find an answer right away.

. . . .

Dr. Kondrot: I agree with you that food is certainly our best medicine. Do you have any favorite products—food products, nutritional products, or detoxification products—that you recommend to your patients?

Dr. Kotulski: People have all kinds of issues with food sensitivities, and that's a whole other discussion. If somebody comes in with advanced cancer, and it has metastasized, I'll give a list of what I call antiangiogenic foods. This will include berries, turmeric, other spices, and fresh and mixed greens. Those are some of my favorites. I recommend asparagus to increase glutathione. Garlic, onion, and cabbage are all great foods as well. We emphasize organic food.

As far as products, we look for clean products that have been tested. In doing nutritional medicine for over 20 years, I've come to favor certain product lines. We'll use those because our clients need to have results. They need to have enhanced vitality, so I'm more inclined to use products that have proven to me that they get a result.

With supplements, I make sure we're doing things that enhance mitochondrial function, like lipoic acid, CoQ10, and things that will increase fatty acid metabolism. We'll use carnitine. We'll do things to enhance detoxification in the bigger sense. We'll talk about amino acids and protein supplements. There are many different detoxification pathways that can be enhanced by supplements.

We put some people on vitamin C protocols, and we use vitamin C in the various forms to impact all parts of the body. The various forms include lyposomal vitamin C to increase intracellular levels, vitamin C palmitate to enhance extracellular levels, and vitamin C in the ascorbate form to work in the gut.

Our clinic is well known for its intravenous treatments. We use a variety of nutrients. We can turn somebody who's in a critical condition around very quickly. In the cases where people are failing fast, we'll use IV nutrition to help them recover.

· ·

Dr. Kondrot: What foods remove heavy metals from the body?

Dr. Kotulski: I mentioned asparagus for upregulating glutathione if you're in that pre-toxification phase. To enhance lymphatic flow, organic celery and beets help with that. To bind toxins, there are things like cilantro. Sometimes we use specific binders. You need to have enhanced fiber at times to get proper elimination of the toxins. If toxins are not bound, they're not getting into the gut and eliminated through the stool; then it's all for naught. The toxins get recycled. Therefore, I err on the side that more is better regarding fibers and may use some calcium glucarate as well to enhance binding.

To expand a little bit, if someone has an active cancer that's metastasized and is well advanced, we'll stress a ketogenic diet. If someone is in a recovery mode, we may go more Mediterranean and more phytonutrients, and not so much animal flesh for protein, if any. We have no one diet; it's very individualized.

. . . .

Dr. Kondrot: Can you explain what a ketogenic diet is and why you would prescribe it?

Dr. Kotulski: There's a lot of misunderstanding with a ketogenic diet. Some people think of the Atkins diet with high protein and high fat. We try to make it a little more nutritionally sound. I reserve the ketogenic for somebody who has an aggressive cancer. One of the important things that must be done when that's the scenario is that you have to change the substrate, the fuel for the cancer. Cancer thrives on glucose. The ketogenic diet will basically turn the glucose fuel line off for cancer, and you'll start burning fat. You break down protein. You may get some glucose from that, but we want to preserve protein in the body so that doesn't happen. We make sure we prescribe supplementation to promote the ketotic state the patient should be in. We get very scientific. We'll monitor with ketotic strips. We'll make sure the patient stays in a relative state of ketosis—not too extreme. We don't want to put them into a coma, obviously.

Glucose is a nutrient that does not need to come in through food. Sometimes this is a major change from what a person is used to eating—additional protein and healthy fat, limiting the majority of their carbohydrates, perhaps no fruit at all, and for sure, no processed sugars of any sort is the goal. This is done for one reason only, to allow the body to recover and to eliminate nutrients going to the cancer. We'll do things to promote anti-angiogenesis that are a little more specific. Certain foods and fluids, like green tea, bok choy, kale, ginseng, mushrooms, and dark chocolate with minimal to no sugar allow the person to recover a little bit.

People on special diets in our office are always transitioning. No one with cancer is ever stuck on any one diet for any significant length of time. The body is either ill or not doing well, or it's in recovery. We like to take the momentum of recovery and make changes accordingly with the diet to promote just that.

. . . .

Dr. Kondrot: Please give us some key takeaway points.

Dr. Kotulski: Being mindful is the number-one thing. If you can appreciate that there are choices with the air you breathe, the water you drink, and the food you consume, you can make a dramatic difference for yourself and the next generation. We have to value health. Right now we value sickness. If you value health, you choose to spend a little more money on food. If you value sickness, you can't afford to eat healthy.

Sherry Rogers, author of *Detoxify or Die*, points this out for anyone who has Stage 4 cancer. In the big scheme of things, you have to be spiritually connected. Your belief system is paramount to any kind of recovery. Feel confident in your belief system and feel grounded with it. Appreciate that it's not you by yourself. There is a higher power, and there is power around you that governs your health. You have to appreciate that as well.

Third, you have to be on your toes at all times when it comes to detoxification. This is not something you get to play with every now and then and do a little detox ten days out of the year. Detoxification should be done on a daily basis. Appreciate the foods that help you detoxify. Perhaps you need to find physicians who can help you detoxify in a more concentrated way. You have to detoxify if you're going to thrive.

The final takeaway point, one more time, is being mindful of all the choices around you. If we're going to promote health for the next generation, we need to be proactive not just with our own choices but also get other people motivated. It's more than finding our healing on an individual path. It's working with those around us if we're going to make the biggest health gains.

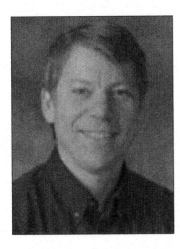

Jeffrey J. Kotulski, DO
Between the Bridges Healing Center
45 Teton Lane
Mankato, MN 56001- 4814
507-388-7488

FIND A HOLISTIC DENTIST AND PRESERVE YOUR HEALTH

Interview with
Carl McMillan, DMD

Dr. Carl McMillan's primary focus for over 20 years has been on holistic dentistry. As a testament to his firm belief in practicing holistic dentistry, Dr. McMillan is a charter member of the International Academy of Mercury Free Dentists (IAMFD) and a member and director of the International Academy of Oral Medicine and Toxicology (IAOMT). These two academies are primarily composed of physicians, dentists, and research scientists who are dedicated to practicing evidence-based health care.

His belief that total body wellness starts in the mouth is the foundation of his practice. Dedicating himself to practicing dentistry according to the principle of "First, do no harm," Dr. McMillan ardently believes in providing his patients with dental care that improves their overall health. Dr. McMillan offers services such as holistic dentistry, cosmetic dentistry, family dentistry, oral sedation, bridges, veneers, crowns, and teeth whitening.

    1. The second most toxic element known to man— mercury—is leaching out of those so-called silver amalgam fillings. I call them mercury fillings, and they're poisoning us.

2. **Studies have been done that show a connection between root canals and some cancers, particularly breast cancer. There's also been an association with MS.**

. . . .

Dr. Kondrot: Please tell us a little bit about your background. Since you're the only dentist featured in this book. I'm sure the readers will be interested in how the dental profession is concerned about heavy metal poisoning and detoxification.

Dr. McMillan: My background is really simple. I meandered through high school and didn't know what I was going to do. I decided to go to college to be an engineer. I started a math and engineering degree and decided I would throw in a little biology.

As I progressed through college and biology particularly, I decided that I wanted to go into the health field. My interest in medicine and health stemmed from growing up as a pretty rambunctious boy. I shot myself with a BB gun when I was ten years old and lost vision in my right eye. I broke a lot of bones. I always knew that I healed fast, and I resisted traditional treatment. If I got a cold or something, I would get so fearful of getting medication that I would pack a little bag and run off to the woods beside our house and hide in the woods to prevent taking medication.

After the accident, they wanted to enucleate my eye, and I said, "No, we're not doing that." I was ten years old. How loud can a ten-year-old boy scream? I was screaming pretty loudly, "No, don't take my eye."

In my junior year at the College of Charleston, I really wanted to be an eye surgeon because I had learned so much about eyes from shooting myself and from all the surgeries I had. I had closed-angle glaucoma, cataract, lens removed and replaced, and several procedures to control glaucoma.

I got an interview at MUSC medical school. I did well on the MCAT. When I told them I wanted to be an ophthalmologist, all three of the interviewers told me I would never be accepted into an ophthalmology program because of having mon- ocular vision. I said, "I don't want to do anything else in medicine. I'll go to dental school." I applied to dental school and got in. They challenged me on whether I would be able to do dentistry with one eye.

My standard answer to that, and even to the physicians who interviewed me for ophthalmology, was "I've played high school baseball and basketball and had no trouble. I excelled at both of those with one eye." Both of those are very depth-perception-oriented sports. I felt like I could do anything I wanted to do.

I was a brash almost-20-year-old when I started dental school. I started out with a couple of minor courses in the summer, and one of those was on dental materials. One of the very first things the professor of that course put up on the blackboard was a formula for amalgam, mercury fillings. Again, I was a brash young guy, and I immediately said, "There is no way you can put five cations together and call them a stable compound. It can't happen, particularly with mercury being liquid at room temperature." I was called to the dean's office and told that if I wanted to make it through dental school, I should sit down, shut up, and learn what I was supposed to learn. So I did. I got brainwashed. I let myself slip into that feeling of "It's hard. All this must be locked in."

I excelled in my class, got out of dental school, and started practicing traditionally. I placed thousands of amalgams. I started recognizing a few things that made me uneasy again, particularly working on one pregnant woman, putting mercury in her mouth because she had a mouthful of decay. I learned that within a year of her child being born, her child was pretty severely neurodevelopmentally mentally delayed. I said, "I have to stop using mercury fillings."

Fast forward just a little bit and I still hadn't stopped at that point. I had two boys, one born in 1990 and one in 1993. My 1993-born son, Collin, at about 19 months all of a sudden reversed his developmental progress. He stopped speaking and participating with his friends in daycare. He started crying and being a little more agitated and clingy. He was not resting as well.

I started searching, and ultimately I was led to mercury again. I said, "What? He's never had mercury." As I dug through that, I found out about vaccinations. He had had his third set of vaccinations at 16 months, just a couple of months before we noticed this significant reversal in his development.

I decided to take him to a friend of mine to do a chelation challenge test on this little 34-pound boy, and his mercury level was 53 micrograms of mercury per liter of urine. I was beside myself. His mom had mercury fillings. The more I learned, the more I felt like the contributing factor had to be vaccines. He didn't crawl around in my dental office. He didn't have any mercury fillings.

At the same time, my mother-in-the-law was diagnosed with early onset Alzheimer's at 56 years old. We took her to a physician at Duke University who was one of the leading authorities on Alzheimer's. He did his testing battery and said, "Absolutely, yes. It's early onset Alzheimer's. We'll do medications until she slips past the usefulness of the medications. Then you'll have to institutionalize her." That was completely against what I believed for family, or anyone else for that matter.

I went to one of my colleagues who is a biological dentist. I said, "Do you know this doctor at Duke?" He said, "Oh, yes. We're very good friends." I said, "Mike, does he know about heavy metals and neurodegenerative diseases?" Mike said, "Of course he does." I said, "When I questioned him on it, he said that has nothing to do with it." Mike looked at me and said, "Carl, if he admitted that he knew heavy metals contribute to Alzheimer's, there would be no funding for his research."

My mother-in-law passed at 61, after living five years with a rapidly progressive neurodegenerative Alzheimer's type of disorder. We did a chelation challenge on her, and her mercury level was in the 240s. That was done through Doctor's Data, a reference being three or less for an adult male or female.

This was all in 1998. At that point, I made the decision to stop using amalgam and start learning as much as I could about detoxification and how to prevent injury in my office to patients and staff. I got involved with the IAOMT, the International Academy of Oral Medicine and Toxicology. I devoured as much information as I could from them. I studied with Hal Huggins three different times for two weeks up in Montreal. From there, I started employing what I considered to be safe protocols to protect patients from exposure to mercury, particularly when amalgams were being removed for replacement, crowning, and/or extraction of teeth. That's what led me to where I am today.

Dr. Kondrot: Mercury in amalgams is something that is actually a leading contributor to many chronic diseases and neurological problems. What do you think patients need to know if they have silver fillings? What should they do?

Dr. McMillan: That's a great question. I don't think there's one answer to that question. First and foremost, I would say that the average public needs to understand that amalgams contain 50 to 54 percent mercury. It's the major component of amalgams. For most everything else in our lives and the industrialized world, we call them by their major component, but we've been lied to about this. This material has been called silver fillings and amalgam to cover up the fact that they have mercury. We know that mercury leaches off of amalgam mercury fillings 24/7. It increases with heat and physical stimulation, whether from chewing, grinding our teeth, brushing our teeth, or having the hygienist polish our teeth.

The average person is being exposed to larger doses than we could get from pounds and pounds of contaminated fish. In 1991, the World Health Organization actually revealed that amalgams contributed five times more mercury to a human being than fish. We need to understand that the second most toxic element known to man, mercury, is leaching out of those so-called silver amalgam fillings. I call them mercury fillings, and they're poisoning us.

Should we all run out and do something about them? I believe we should all limit our toxins. I believe our bodies have a finite ability to handle, process, and dispose of toxins. If someone feels like the mercury might be contributing to their ill health, they should seek a properly trained biological dentist who follows at least minimal protocols to protect them while having the mercury fillings removed.

I can't tell you how many patients I've seen who had their fillings taken out because they were trying to do the right thing proactively. They weren't having any physical problem before, and they suddenly developed many different kinds of health problems. We should do our research as to how it's done safely, where it can be done, and if anything needs to be done to protect the body and promote the body's ability to detox naturally and/or with help before we have our amalgams removed.

Dr. Kondrot: One of the problems I see is that a lot of patients will panic. When they discover they have some mercury amalgams, they run to a dentist who isn't properly trained. They'll get all of their amalgams removed in one sitting, and their health begins to decline. Please describe the protocols that are established for safe removal. Is it necessary to receive some type of ongoing chelation during the process?

Dr. McMillan: I would say that we all need support if we are heavy metal poisoned. Unfortunately, if we're toxic with mercury, we're toxic with other heavy metals too because it shuts our pathways down for dealing with other heavy metals. Often, we'll see people who are toxic with lead, chromium, antimony, nickel, and lots of different heavy metals. Some are more neurologically toxic. Some are more organ toxic. I believe that all toxins build up and are additive, so we absolutely need to have medical support of some sort to help our bodies get ready to detox and to handle any kind of exposure.

That leads to the question you really asked. "Should there be some ongoing chelation and detoxification while they have these mercury fillings?" I'm no expert in this field from a standpoint of chelation. But I can offer this: Why would we stir the pot with a chelator that goes deep into tissues to pull out the heavy metals if we're continually being exposed to them through amalgams and/or other metal restorations in our mouths?

No one has been able to demonstrate to me that there's a safe or unsafe approach to that with scientific numbers. Knowing what most of the chelators do and talking to my friend, Boyd Haley, a biochemist and developer of what I believe will be the very best heavy metal—and particularly mercury—chelator, I don't believe we should heavily chelate people unless their exposure is removed.

Dr. Kondrot: My approach is to advise patients to have their mercury amalgams removed slowly and then have some type of ongoing chelation done. I think that no matter how careful a dentist is in removing amalgams, some mercury and toxic substances are going to be leached into the body.

Dr. McMillan: I think you're right. Even with all the protocols, there's potential for some exposure. But I believe that with the protocols we currently follow, there's less exposure than patients get daily from the fillings being in their mouths.

The protocols are different with all the different groups that promote safe removal of mercury. That's one of my frustrations. There's no consistency. We're trying to build that consistency by having a minimum protocol dentists should use, but I don't think there should be minimum standards. We should use every protocol feasible to protect patients, staff, and the atmosphere.

First of all, we have the patient take some activated charcoal before the procedure, rinse, and swallow. We place a rubber dam made of nitrile inside the mouth. Latex is non-protective; it's like a sheer curtain to the sun. Mercury passes right through it. It's important to use a nitrile rubber dam to isolate an area of the mouth.

The patient has a separate breathing source, and the dentist and assistant have either a separate breathing source or a mercury vapor mask to protect them. We have full-face coverage for the patient and full-body coverage down to their ankles with a plastic-backed paper covering. We use high-volume suction, high volumes of water, and suction behind the rubber dam.

I remove amalgams by the chunk method—taking them out in big chunks versus grinding them out. Grinding is the worst thing we can do for amalgams. Once we have it all out, we chelate the tooth and rinse it. Then we have the patient rinse again with activated charcoal and swallow. The patient then goes to their physician for an IV vitamin C and any chelation they recommend. That's where your knowledge comes in. I work with some physicians who do what they call mild chelation while we're removing the amalgams.

. . . .

Dr. Kondrot: I think it's really important that people go to a dentist who is properly trained. Just like in all professions, some people may take a weekend course and become an expert. Are there certain dental organizations that certify or have extensive training so a consumer knows the dentist is properly trained?

Dr. McMillan: Yes. There are a couple of them. The most well-known and the one that, in my opinion, does the most research into techniques and protocols for safe removal is the International Academy of Oral Medicine and Toxicology. I sit on the board for the IAOMT, and I'm the chair of the education committee. We oversee the protocols that we recommend for safe removal. To become an accredited member, one has to demonstrate that they follow the protocols necessary to protect the patient, staff, and environment. That's called an accreditation.

Then there's the Holistic Dental Association. They follow our protocols. There's the Biological Dentistry and Medicine Academy. They follow our protocols with a little of Hal Huggins' protocol added in, particularly paying attention to the electrical activity of metal fillings. Those are the three main groups. I've stated this to my physician friends. I would love to tie the chelating doctors in with the IAOMT so we can come to a good scientific consensus on whether chelation should happen before all amalgams are removed, during, after, and at what levels.

. . . .

Dr. Kondrot: Can you tell us the bad news about root canals?

Dr. McMillan: Root canals are the standard of care in dentistry for saving a dead tooth, whether that tooth dies because of an abscess or trauma.

What is a root canal? It's the cleansing of the inside main root canal system. It's the cleansing of dead tissue and bacteria and then filling that space with a filling material. Often that filling material is gutta-percha (a form of natural rubber). In the biological dentistry world, there have been some materials called Biocalax and Endocal-10 used instead of the gutta-percha.

Really, the material is not the problem. Although we could talk about the toxins and the potential there, the real problem is that a tooth is not a solid mass. It is a very porous mass that forms tiny micro dentinal tubules that go in every direction inside the root structure and dentin up into the crown of the tooth. That tubule system is meant as a passageway for nutrients to the tooth and as long as there is a neurovascular bundle inside the tooth. In other words, the tooth is alive; there is a pumping of fluids through that tubule system.

When that tooth gets infected and dies, there's no longer that positive pump inside the tooth. The bacteria that live in our mouths are both good and bad, but as the tooth dies, it becomes an anaerobic environment. As we know, the bad bugs in life are the anaerobes, and those bugs migrate in and through all those dentinal tubules. When the root canal is done, the tubules can't be cleansed. They are too small for our instruments or our cleaning solutions. The most traditional standard solution is sodium hypochlorite, bleach. Ozone has also been used.

Ozone has a lot of promise, but in the root canal realm, I don't believe it can penetrate all the tubules because it breaks down way too fast. In a molar, for instance, there's somewhere between 12 and 16 miles of dentinal tubules, so there's no way it can be completely sterilized. Even if they could be sterilized, there's no positive pump. The bacteria from around the tooth in the periodontal ligament space can march right in, set up shop, and produce their toxins.

Weston A. Price, a dentist and researcher, performed studies with his team in the late 1890s and early 1900s. He did this research for the ADA (American Dental Association) on root canals. They produced a 1,167-page report on the pitfalls of root canals and the bugs that were being found in those root canal teeth. Their research, but primarily his research, included removing root canal teeth from people with all kinds of degenerative diseases and finding that their health improved.

First, they cultured them to see which bugs grew. There were a lot of anaerobic bugs. Virulent endotoxin-producing anaerobes grew. Not only that, but they cut these teeth up into little pieces and implanted them under the skin of rabbits and guinea pigs and reproduced some of those diseases.

We could argue today that our techniques are so much better and that we do a better job cleaning and disinfecting the root canals, so the teeth are okay. Hal Huggins along with a good friend of mine, Dr. Stuart Nunnally, did research in modern times. They did this along with Boyd Haley at the University of Kentucky. They extracted root canal teeth that patients wanted out, but they didn't extract them until they had them evaluated by root canal specialists called endodontists who agreed that the tooth looked fine on X-ray.

They took these teeth out, put them in an anaerobic medium and sent them off to Boyd Haley, and he did research on the toxins that were being produced.

Those toxins were more toxic to the enzymatic systems tested from the body than was mercury. He started off with a 1:10 dilution, and that was so strong it blew all the enzyme systems off his chromatography gel. Then he diluted it down 1:100. Ultimately, he went to 1:1000 to get it to work with the chromatography gel. Root canals are at least as toxic for us as mercury. Like I tell my patients, it's about toxic load. All of them add to our toxic load.

· ·

Dr. Kondrot: Can you mention the association of root canals to some serious diseases, like cancer, and what studies have been done to support that theory?

Dr. McMillan: I can speak in generalities. I know studies have been done that connect root canals and some cancers, particularly breast cancer. I think we're actually going to find an association with many others. There's also been a link with MS.

· ·

Dr. Kondrot: We've covered a lot of really important material. Do you have any closing words for the readers of this chapter?

Dr. McMillan: First and foremost, we need to advocate for ourselves, even if people don't believe that heavy metals or root canals could be contributing to our disease process. We have to be our own advocates and seek out those who are willing to help us with safe alternatives and help us find as much information as required to make the decisions we need to make for our own personal health. We need to seek out doctors who are knowledgeable in heavy metal detoxification and chelation to support the body to heal itself.

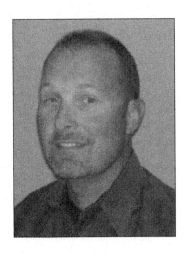

Carl McMillan, DMD, PA
Holistic Dental Centers
www.smilesraleigh.com

20905 Torrence Chapel Road, Suite 201-202
Cornelius, NC 28031
704-765-3150

218 Ashville Avenue, Suite 30
Cary, NC 27518
919-865-0700

NEW DIAGNOSTIC AND TREATMENT APPROACHES TO DETOXIFICATION

Interview with
Dorothy F. Merritt, MD

Dorothy Merritt, MD, is certified by the American Board of Internal Medicine and has been practicing medicine in the Galveston County area for more than 22 years. She is dedicated to the health of that community.

Dr. Merritt was raised in Kansas and attended medical school at the University of Kansas. She completed her internal medicine training at Baylor College of Medicine in Houston, TX. She has been active in developing programs that maximize health and wellness while identifying and treating environmentally caused illnesses. Dr. Merritt uses many natural approaches to prevention of illness and integrates them into her primary care practice.

1. **Those born between 1925 -1975 have significant exposure to lead via lead stored in their bones. About one-third will be okay, but two-thirds will have conditions ranging from hypertension to atherosclerosis.**

2. **People born after 1980 should have such low buildup of bone lead that heart conditions due to lead**

accumulation will be almost obsolete.

3. **Detoxification requires a comprehensive approach:**

    a. All elimination pathways must be open: sweat, bowels, and urine.

    b. Water-soluble chemicals and fat-bound toxins need specific protocols.

    c. Metal detoxification requires specialized compounds.

. . . .

Dr. Kondrot: Please tell us a little bit about your background.

Dr. Merritt: I am a board certified internist (University of Kansas and Baylor College of Medicine) who has practiced medicine in Texas City, Texas, for the last 28 years. I have successfully integrated numerous therapies that reduce the cost of medical care and increase good health outcomes. I integrate foods that support detoxification, supplements that override genetic SNPs (Single Nucleotide Polymorphism) that hinder the detoxification process, and check for environmental exposures that are common in my area, such as solvents and lead. Starting interventions such as EDTA chelation and glutathione builders early on is the key to preventing long-term disease. Recently, I was a principal investigator for TACT (Trial to Assess Chelation Therapy)—the landmark EDTA chelation research project that showed a 26 to 58 percent decrease in death, bypass surgery, and hospitalization in a post heart attack population of adults 50 years or older. I co-authored the latest TACT publication on a diabetic subgroup, which showed 58 percent benefit to those treated with EDTA (*Circulation*, November 2014). The study also showed a 43 percent reduction in death rates in diabetics who had a heart attack previous to the study.

I lecture new students of chelation at ACAM (American College for Advancement in Medicine) and ICIM (International College of Integrative Medicine). I developed an academically based protocol applicable to individuals born between

1925 and 1975. With it, we can decide who should be treated now because of lifelong lead exposure before a major catastrophe like stroke or heart attack occurs.

. . . .

Dr. Kondrot: How did you become interested in integrative medicine?

Dr. Merritt: I came out of training as a typical internal medicine specialist, but after the first year of seeing the same diseases over and over, I knew I needed to understand the causes better and put in interventions community-wide to prevent these problems. I was put on the board of public health and studied the disease trends in my area. When I did a nutritional assay called SpectraCell, which measures the intracellular level of vitamins, minerals, and antioxidants, I found out that my patients were deficient in all of these as well as deficient in an amino acid called cysteine and a tripeptide called glutathione. These are the preliminary substances to the master antioxidants in the body. They are needed for the removal of normal products of metabolism as well as toxins and for repair of tissues.

I became the medical director of hospice for my area, and it was an eye opening experience when I gave the patients a simple vitamin supplement and 600mg NAC (N-Acetyl Cysteine) daily. They lived 18 days longer in less pain and felt better. The pharmacy costs went down 50 percent immediately. Imagine what would happen if I gave it to my general population of patients. I did and what happened was a 90 percent reduction in admissions to the hospital; insurance companies started calling and wanting to know if they could buy my "disease management system." What followed was a journey of education on nutrition that led to EDTA chelation and a simple, science-based plan to keep people healthier.

. . . .

Dr. Kondrot: What important things do people need to know about detoxification?

Dr. Merritt: There are four main areas to consider:

First, in order for detoxification to occur, all elimination pathways must be open: sweat, bowels, and urine. Normal products of metabolism as well as toxicants need to be moved out of the body so that the body doesn't back up like a sewer. If you try to remove too many too fast, it is like the 5:00 p.m. rush hour in any city. Sweating in an infrared sauna is good, but exercising is good too. I once had a patient with high metal toxicity. He told tell me that after he mowed a big field in the summer heat, his liver area would not hurt for three days and he felt better. Since he was unemployed and disabled from his metal grinding job, I told him to mow lawns in order to make money as well as to treat himself at the same time.

Second, you have to know how to detox water-soluble chemicals as well as fat-bound toxins. The common fat-bound toxins are pesticides, dioxins, PCBs, and some solvents. These go from fat to liver to gallbladder and are dumped out in the intestine where 90 percent are reabsorbed downstream in the colon—unless their absorption is blocked. Fiber will bind 25 percent, but about one to two ounces of chips eaten daily containing olestra (brand name Olean) will cause a 3,000 percent increased excretion in the stool daily. Fat biopsies in one study showed that after two years of this treatment, body fat was free of fat-bound toxins that had been measured at the beginning. Although chips are not an ideal vector, the good far outweighs the bad, in my opinion, especially for just two years of chip eating at a low level of one ounce per day. Warning: Do not eat more than two ounces of these chips per day, or you will pay the consequences of malabsorption with diarrhea and cramps.

Third, to clear water-soluble toxins, you need phase one and two pathways open. Glutathione levels need to be elevated and maintained. I tell people to try NAC (N-Acetyl Cysteine) twice a day and take a supplement or eat food that includes antioxidants, minerals, and B vitamins that are already methylated or activated in order to support the liver's processing these toxicants. I always have them take the activated B vitamins due to the large proportion of the United States population that has genetic defects in absorbing these substances. Methyl B12 and methyl folate are not found in nature generally, although barley has a small amount of methyl folate.

Fourth, metal detox has to be done with compounds that bind metals and re-move them from the body. The art of detoxing from metals includes knowing how to get metals out of brain, tissue, blood, and other areas like bone as well as which binders and chelators are indicated. It is also important to know what nutrients to supplement with to prevent problems during cleansing of these toxicants. My mentor, Dr. Walter Crinnion, states that metals are like a "hairball" blocking up the drain. Once you remove these metals, detoxing other substances is easier. This is another way of saying that the metals block up so many metabolic pathways that it is very difficult to maintain these pathways without first removing metal ions that are preventing the various metabolic cycles from working.

. . . .

Dr. Kondrot: What are the major substances we need to detoxify?

Dr. Merritt: In the last 70 years in the United States, we have been exposed to high doses of lead, pesticides, PCBs, solvents, and a whole host of chemicals that we don't know a lot about. Testing performed on human fat and tissue shows hundreds of chemicals that do not belong there. Getting each of these out of the body is important to long-term health.

I did additional environmental medicine training at Southwest College of Naturopathic Medicine with Walter Crinnion, ND, in the early 2000s, and it changed my whole approach to disease as I practice it in my industrially based petrochemical community. Dr. Crinnion's book, *Clean, Lean, and Green,* tells how to use food to turn on the detox systems in the body. It is easy to read, easy to follow, and based in science. Supplements are important but nature provides us with good sources of detoxification in our foods. Once you get the excess chemicals out of your body, carefully selected organic food sources will help maintain the process.

I trained at ACAM 18 years ago, and I now teach the students how to do EDTA chelation. ACAM was the first organization that studied and taught others how to chelate with EDTA, and they have always advocated EDTA as a treatment for coronary heart disease. Lead is still the number one problem in the United States as far as metals are concerned. We polluted the air and the people from 1925 to 1979 with lead fumes from gasoline. The legacy has left us with a population riddled with heart and neurological diseases. Hopefully, the majority of people born after 1980 should have such low exposure and such low buildup of bone lead that their cardiovascular and neurological risk of heart conditions due to lead will be almost negligible.

. . . .

Dr. Kondrot: What is your basic approach to the workup of patients who

come to you for this kind of care?

Dr. Merritt: The first thing I do is take a good history and do a good physical. Then I start patients on a combination of supplements that support the methylation and detoxification pathways in the body. My usual regimen is four to six UltraNutrient capsules daily (Pure Encapsulations) and N-Acetyl Cysteine 600mg twice a day (for most), and we have discussions about diet, sauna, exercise, and metal testing. I do a blood lead level in addition to other labs, and I suggest a chelation challenge with pre and post urine samples to look for metal burdens in the body.

. . . .

Dr. Kondrot: What unique advanced testing do you have in your office?

Dr. Merritt: I have a number of new unique testing systems in my office, and I choose the appropriate ones for each patient. My ESTek Body Scanner screens for about 200 physiological parameters of the whole body. I measure these repeatedly over time to monitor improvements. It is inexpensive ($100) and is quick and reproducible. If you are tired, I can determine the cause of your fatigue. Perhaps your adrenals and thyroid glands are not working properly, or your autonomic nervous system is dysfunctional; perhaps you are depressed, or you may have some other condition causing fatigue. I have a MCG (multichannel cardiogram) from Premier Heart that is about as good as a heart catheterization but, in only eight minutes, tells us much more in a noninvasive manner and is less expensive ($300). I can measure blood flow during and after chelation and show that the chelation is increasing heart blood flow immediately during the first treatment. It is good to monitor the effect of other cardiac therapies or lifestyle changes too. I have equipment that measures the electrical gut and detects different types of irritable bowel syndrome (IBS). I have a Nexalin machine that resets the brain's limbic and hypothalamus system and restores serotonin, dopamine, and norepinephrine without medications in just ten treatments. Many toxic people get the toxins out and then still feel tired. Resetting the hypothalamus is the key to restoring vitality in these people.

. . . .

Dr. Kondrot: Who do you recommend have EDTA chelation?

Dr. Merritt: I just finished an analysis of all the literature on lead and bone levels that cause disease. Fortunately, the levels of lead in the blood have diminished with our national efforts to limit exposure. However, 90 percent of the previous exposure level is in our bones and comes out ten times faster between ages 40 to 80. This means we are our own source of toxicity. All people born from 1925 to 1975 have significant exposure to lead through that stored in their bones. About one third will be okay, but two thirds will have conditions of their vascular system ranging from hypertension to atherosclerosis. They may also have neurological disorders and kidney dysfunction that can be directly related to the lead in their bones. Even 44 percent of all cataracts are attributed to lifetime exposure and storage of lead in the bones.

The Normative Aging Studies done at the National Institutes of Health (NIH) as well as the CDC's NHANES (National Health and Nutrition Examination Survey) studies of blood lead levels since the 1970s have shown that lead causes increased vascular disease and death in the form of strokes, hypertension, heart attacks, and peripheral vascular disease. They have also shown lead causes people to have more osteoporosis, walk slower, lose more teeth, have kidney problems, have shrunken brain tissue, and a whole host of neurocognitive and psychiatric conditions.

I have come up with a protocol to treat these people (if they need it) before they become visibly ill by using my body scan vascular measurements, a blood lead level, age, and inventory of current complaints. I also believe the saying, "It's not the germ that the problem; it's the terrain." This means we need to make your body's defense systems strong and resistant to the lead or toxicants you have left in your tissue, while at the same time minimizing new exposure.

We know definitively from the TACT trial that EDTA chelation is safe. We know that ischemic heart disease costs $350 billion a year to treat. In EDTA, we have a proven therapy that is inexpensive, and reduces death, rehospitalization, and bypass surgery by up to 58 percent in certain populations like diabetics, in addition to "standard of care" medications. Hopefully, after TACT 2, the FDA will approve EDTA as an indicated treatment for vascular disease in addition to its FDA approved use for lead toxicity.

In the meantime, patients can do EDTA chelation under an alternative medicine practitioner and pay cash, or they can sign up for the upcoming TACT trial if they are diabetic, have had a previous heart attack, are 50 years or older, and have kidneys that work. It will be a randomized controlled trial, so there is a 50 percent chance they will get treatment and a 50 percent chance of placebo. The trial should start in late 2015 or when funded.

(Editor's note: www.clinicaltrials.gov may be a good place to look for this opportunity, but TACT 2 is not listed as of this writing.)

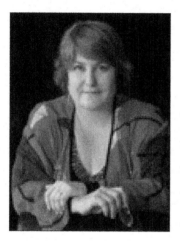

Dorothy Merritt, MD
Mainland Primary Care Physicians
6807 Emmett F. Lowry Expressway,
Suite 103
Texas City, TX 77591
409-938-1770
www.mpcptexas.com (practice websit)
www.SWWellness.com (website for articles)

FOR OPTIMUM HEALTH, YOU NEED A STRATEGY

Interview with
David Minkoff, MD

Dr. David Minkoff graduated from the University of Wisconsin Medical School in 1974 and was elected to the prestigious Alpha Omega Alpha Honors Medical Fraternity for very high academic achievement. He then worked for more than 20 years in the area of traditional medicine before making the switch to alternative medicine when he and his wife, Sue, founded LifeWorks Wellness Center in Clearwater, Florida. LifeWorks is now one of this country's foremost alternative health clinics, offering a wide range of cutting-edge protocols.

In 2000, Dr. Minkoff founded BodyHealth, a nutrition company that offers a range of unique dietary supplements to the public and practitioners. BodyHealth's mission is to educate doctors and the public with information to improve the body's condition and supply the products needed to do that.

Dr. Minkoff is passionate about fitness and is a 41-time Ironman finisher, including eight appearances at the Ironman World Championships in Hawaii. He also writes two weekly newsletters, The Optimum Health Report *and the* BodyHealth Fitness Newsletter.

1. **What we found is that almost every person who has chronic illness has high levels of heavy metals: mercury, arsenic, lead, or cadmium. We're seeing more uranium because of the fallout from the Gulf War and Fukushima.**

2. **If you have a chronic problem like hypertension, high cholesterol, obesity, diabetes, cancer, autoimmune disease, osteoporosis, or fatigue, modern medicine doesn't help you.**

. . . .

Dr. Kondrot: Please tell us a little bit about your medical training and how you became interested in chelation and detoxification.

Dr. Minkoff: I decided at a very young age that I wanted to be a doctor. I think I was about five years old. I had two uncles who were doctors, and, for some reason, that seemed like the career path for me. I went to medical school at the University of Wisconsin. I was the first language major who made it into medical school at that time. I didn't know what I wanted to do in medicine. I was very torn, so I decided to do a rotating internship. I went to Mercy Hospital in San Diego, California, which is one of the hospitals in the University of California San Diego Center. I did a rotating internship for a year, and my first rotation was pediatrics. After a couple of months my instructor said, "Boy, you'd be a really good pediatrician." I thought, "Maybe I should be a pediatrician," so I decided to be a pediatrician and work with kids. I'd been a camp counselor and lifeguard, and I'd always worked with kids. After my third year of residency, they appointed me to chief resident, and I ran the teaching program at UCSD for a year.

I still didn't know exactly what I wanted to do, so I did a fellowship in infectious disease. Under their tutelage I had a very interesting two-year fellowship there. My research project was working with new antiviral drugs, acyclovir and ribavirin. Both are still in use today. For the next ten years, I had a busy life. I had a general pediatrics practice; I was co-director of a neonatal intensive care unit; I consulted in the hospital for adult and pediatric infectious disease cases; I was infection control officer at a community hospital; and was an attending physician at the Pediatric Infectious Disease department at UCSD. For variety, I had a moonlighting job on weekends doing emergency medicine in a busy trauma ER, and with that, a wife and three kids, and training for Ironman triathlons; life couldn't have been more interesting.

I started my infectious disease career right at the beginning of the AIDS epidemic, so we were seeing a lot of cases that were complicated and unusual. It was also a time when a lot of the Hmong people from Southeast Asia had come to California, and they had a lot of exotic parasitic diseases, which was very interesting. I learned a lot.

In 1990, we relocated to Clearwater, Florida, where I took a sabbatical for six months to do some personal enhancement training. After the sabbatical, the family was really happy in Clearwater, and we decided to stay. I got a job there in an emergency room.

In 1997, my wife, who was a very good triathlete and who always took care of herself, took vitamins, ate really well, maintained a good body weight, and all this stuff, decided she didn't like the way the silver fillings in her teeth looked. She went to a dentist who was supposedly a mercury-free dentist, and he took the fillings out of her teeth—improperly.

Within six weeks, she was sick. She got thyroiditis. She woke up one morning and couldn't even lift her arm to brush her teeth. Also, her gluteus maximus muscle on one side didn't work. I thought, "Oh, my God! What is this?" I had her see the best doctors I knew, and they didn't know what she had. They said, "This is some kind of autoimmune disease. It might be multiple sclerosis." I said, "What do you do for that?" There weren't really any good treatments.

She's a nurse, and she runs a home health nursing agency. A new practitioner had moved into her office complex. On the marquee, it said "Natural Dentistry." One night I was picking her up, and he came walking out of his office toward the car, and I introduced myself to him. I said, "I'm an ER doctor, and my wife developed this new neurological problem shortly after she had her mercury fillings removed. Could these two things be related? He said, "Yes, they sure could be, but you're not going to find anybody who will even put that on their differential diagnosis. You'd better learn about it. The guy who knows the most about it is in Seattle. You'd better take some courses from him. You have to learn some energy medicine and muscle testing, or you'll never figure it out."

Not knowing what else to do, I went to Seattle, got trained, came home, and tested her. Lo and behold, she had high levels of mercury, not only on the energetic testing but also on the challenged urine testing. I thought this was pretty amazing medicine and that it could help a lot of people. So I set up a part-time practice in the back of her nursing agency, and we started to treat her. Meanwhile, my wife, who had always been interested in alternative medicine, dragged me to every seminar that Jeffrey Bland—renowned biochemist and a leader in the fields of functional medicine, nutritional medicine, and systems biology—ever offered, and a lot of other places. I learned a lot about nutritional biochemistry, detoxification, and functional medicine.

When I looked around for treatments for my wife for the toxic mercury levels, there was very little to work with. As I pursued solutions, I met a research bio-chemist and, together, we created a product that was an oral chelator. It not only bound mercury but also lead, arsenic, uranium, and aluminum. It was in the form of a sublingual spray and absorbed well through mucous membranes. It consists of some very unique peptides that form very tight bonds with metals that are excreted in the stool. We called this product Metal-Free, because that is what it did for the body. After my wife started taking it, her levels started to come down and within six months she was feeling great, and all signs of toxicity were gone.

With her success, I started testing other patients who had illnesses like MS, Parkinson's, chronic fatigue, and autoimmune diseases. To my surprise, I found that nearly all of them had high levels of heavy metals. As we began to treat them, they responded just as my wife did, and we had great success. My little office grew and grew, and pretty soon we needed another space. We went from the one room to a bigger space. Then we went from the bigger space to the office complex we have now, and Lifeworks Wellness Center was born.

As we went along, we learned a lot more about how to help somebody get better. What we found is that almost every person who has chronic illness has high levels of heavy metals: mercury, arsenic, lead, cadmium, or a combination of the above. These days we're seeing more and more uranium because of the fallout from the Gulf War and Fukushima. With the high levels of heavy metal contamination in the environment, people accumulate these things, and they don't let them go very easily. These metals are toxic. They block all kinds of energy reactions and enzyme reactions in the body. Unless we can help people detoxify their heavy metals, a lot of people won't get better.

At LifeWorks Wellness Center, I work with a naturopath, chiropractor, nutritionist, and nurse practitioner. We have really good success, and chelation is one of the cornerstones of what we do.

. . . .

Dr. Kondrot: That was a profound story. As a physician, it feels terrible to be helpless when someone near and dear to you develops an illness.

Dr. Minkoff: What's amazing is that most doctors' stable view on reality is that if they don't know about it, they don't like it. I was like that too, but I went to the seminars, started to learn, and saw incredible doctors getting good results. I could see that this made a lot of sense.

What I was doing in the emergency room would help people. If you get hit by a car, have a heart attack, have a kidney stone, or your appendix bursts, modern medicine can be very effective. If you have a chronic problem like hypertension, high cholesterol, obesity, diabetes, cancer, autoimmune disease, osteoporosis, or fatigue, modern medicine doesn't help you. They're going to probably end up hurting you because what they do doesn't do anything to fix what is actually wrong and what actually caused the problem in the first place. Chronic illness is not a drug deficiency disease, but that is the way it's treated.

The other thing I wanted to add is that when I moved to San Diego in 1974, Frank Shorter had won the Olympic marathon, and it got me very interested in running. At the same time, my father had a heart attack. I thought, "I'd better do something to help my own health." I started running marathons.

In 1982, *Wide World of Sports* televised the Ironman World Championship from Kona, Hawaii. It inspired me to do the race, which I completed in October 1982. Since that time, I have completed 40 Ironman triathlons with eight of them in Hawaii at the World Championships. In my quest to help others get healthy, I decided I had to be a good example and live right myself. It has worked. At age 66, I can compete in a 13- or 14-hour Ironman race and enjoy it. It's because these therapies, including chelation, make you stronger longer so you can have a healthier life.

. . . .

Dr. Kondrot: To put things into perspective, please describe what is involved with an Ironman triathlon.

Dr. Minkoff: The race is a 2.4-mile swim followed by a 112-mile bike ride followed by a full marathon, 26.2 miles. A professional will do it in a little over eight hours. For somebody my age, 12 to 13 hours is pretty darn good. I've been competing since 1982, and it's a lot of fun. You can't do it if you're fat and sick. You can do it if you eat well, get enough sleep, manage your stress, and take care of yourself. Then you handle your own body's weaknesses. Keeping your vitamins, amino acids, and essential fats in a good range is important.

We live in a toxic environment. On an average day, a person will come in contact with hundreds if not thousands of environmental toxins, chemicals, pesticides, heavy metals, additives and all this junk, so you need to have a strategy to stay healthy. This is not just for athletes but also for the regular person. You need to be able to get this stuff out of your body. It's going to come out through sweat, stool, urine, or breath. People who are sick accumulate it all, and then they get sicker. I have a very busy practice and a busy family life with triathlons thrown in, and I write newsletters on health for about 30,000 people a week, but I find time to take care of myself. I do ozone sauna a couple of times a week. I do infrared sauna almost every day. I'm eating very well, and I'm taking a load of supplements to try to keep my body in good health. I think my patients look to me and notice it, and they're inspired that their doctor isn't the old, fat guy who's telling them one thing and doing another. I try to live it, and I think it inspires them to be able to do it too.

. . . .

Dr. Kondrot: I'm going to start referring to you as the high-performance doctor. You're not only improving your own performance but also helping oth-

ers who are struggling with their health. What is the important information that the general public should know about detoxification and chelation?

Dr. Minkoff: I think people can do low-grade natural detoxification and chelation with over-the-counter types of things without usually getting into trouble. But if you are sick, fatigued, and in pain, you need a good natural doctor. Chances are high that you are full of heavy metals, have mercury in the mouth, root canals, bad periodontal disease, and a high viral load. People have infections floating around their system with Epstein-Barr, cytomegalovirus, Lyme, parasites, and fungi. They're on a high sugar diet. They're overweight. They eat fast food. Their gut doesn't work very well, so they don't absorb nutrients. In fact, in their gut are a few hundred trillion bacteria, which are the wrong kind.

In my experience, I never put those people on an IV chelation program because I have seen them get sicker. We have a way of testing the body to try to get at the autonomic nervous system of the body to guide you in how you get this person from wherever he is to where you want him to go. What we find is that IV chelation or even strong oral chelation is often very close to a last step. I've had so many patients come in and say, "The doctor gave me the IV chelation, and I got sick. I've been sick ever since. I haven't been able to think ever since." It's because it's done in the wrong order.

Yes, chelation is a wonderful therapy. It helps cardiovascular disease and diabetes. It helps detoxify people and restore their energy. If it's done in the wrong order and you are sick, it probably isn't the first thing you should do. You need professional help to figure out the right order of things.

I often will work with someone for three, six, or nine months before we've handled their parasites, viruses, fungi, leaky gut, hormones, and nutritional deficiencies. If you have low magnesium, low selenium, or low zinc levels in your body, and you try to pull mercury, the body won't let it go. It will hold on to that mercury because it's deficient in minerals.

I fix all that stuff first, including hormones. What you get then is a person on a good diet. They've having a good bowel movement or two every day. Their hormone levels are in physiologic range for a younger person. They don't have any deficiencies of minerals, amino acids, or essential fats. Their gut flora is restored. Their teeth are handled, so there aren't any big dental issues that are stressors. What will usually come up on energetic testing at that point is that now your body is ready to handle expelling the mercury, lead, or arsenic. Then we do the chelation.

I do this combination through a couple of IVs a week of what we call chezone, which is ozone plus chelation. It's way better than just EDTA by itself as a chelator. A lot of people still have organisms in their body that shouldn't be in there, so you dissolve the biofilms with the ozone. It kills the bacteria. A lot of the mercury or lead load is in the bacteria or fungi. They dump it. The chelator is right there. You bind it up, and then it goes very smoothly. On the off days, I give them Metal-Free. It's a spray. Another one I developed is called Body Detox. It also handles metals and a lot of biotoxins—toxins from other organisms. With a nutritional program and supplementation, people sail through it. They do really well.

We go slowly. We don't want people to get sick while they're detoxing. I don't believe in this thing called the healing crisis. What really happens in a healing crisis is that the doctor went too fast or you went too fast. We try to get people better and better as they go. I've added another step that some people need. A lot of people have allergies to either the heavy metals themselves or things like sulfur, which are necessary to bind heavy metals. We do an acupressure desensitization procedure so that when these metals are activated during the chelation process, their nervous system doesn't react to it. This is an important part of it, and it makes it go more smoothly.

. . . .

Dr. Kondrot: Please share a story that illustrates why it's important not to rush into chelation early.

Dr. Minkoff: I'm working with a woman now in her mid-40s. She's had six children. She's very fit. She came to me after getting an IV DMPS by another doctor who said she had heavy metals. She does have heavy metals, but she also had everything else that I listed above. The first thing he did with her when she told the story of about three years of severe chronic fatigue is a heavy metal challenge. The doctor collected urine, and she did indeed have very high levels of mercury and lead, so he started her on chelation. After a treatment or two, she couldn't get out of bed or think straight. She was worse, and she didn't know what was wrong. She knew that whatever was being done was not right.

I began to treat her about a year ago, and when we did the energetic testing to find out what the priority was in her body, it turned out that she had a lot of gut issues. She had fungi, parasites, bad bacteria, and leaky gut, and she was auto-immune. It took five or six months to get that straightened out to the point where she could actually eat food and absorb it, and the food wouldn't leak into the rest of her body. She was also hormone deficient and had a lot of Lyme bacteria in her body. We spent eight or nine months treating that stuff. It was somewhat of a roller coaster, but she kept getting better, and her good days increased.

We then desensitized her to sulfur, mercury, and lead along with a few other things. It had a dramatic effect on her health. Within a few days of that, she started to be able to run. We now have her on an oral chelation program with Metal-Free and Body Detox with some chlorella, and she's doing marvelously.

That's a typical story of someone I see. I'm not in a hurry. I want to build a platform of health underneath. We will be starting her on IV chelation in the next week or two because I think now she can actually handle it. We'll get rid of the heavy metals, and she'll go off into the sunset and be fine. It's taken almost a year before we started the chelation phase.

. . . .

Dr. Kondrot: Do you have another patient story to illustrate this?

Dr. Minkoff: I deal with quite a few high-performance athletes. I do some podcasts and a newsletter that goes out every other week to athletes. About 30,000 athletes get the *BodyHealth Performance* newsletter. A lot of athletes consult me because they want performance, and they don't feel good. I had an athlete in the local area who is a triathlete, and the problem with many triathletes is that they tend to train too much. He was exercising more than he could recover, and his testosterone level was about 75. It should be 800, 900, or 1,000. His cortisol levels were very low all day, and his DHEA levels were very low. He had a lot of muscle aches and pains. When I first saw him and tested him, it showed that he had a parasitic infestation that needed to be addressed first.

The next thing we found is that he had a really severe amino acid deficiency. His gut was so torn up from parasites, and he was very gluten intolerant, but he didn't know it. We got him on a Paleo diet. He's off gluten, dairy, beans, and processed foods. He only eats real foods. Then we tuned up his gut and got rid of the parasite. We balanced his hormones, and he started to feel better and better.

Then he had a very high lead issue. We did oral chelation with Metal-Free and Body Detox and IV EDTA on him with glutathione and ozone, which was the chezone. He's back competing. He feels great. He's the star in his age group. He actually has real health now. Before, the training ran him down because his body couldn't recover because it had so many other toxic things going on.

· ·

Dr. Kondrot: What do you advise patients to do right now to improve their health?

Dr. Minkoff: It's probably 90 percent lifestyle. What does that mean? They need to eat the right foods, and not too much, to get their body weight ideal, and their blood sugar less than 90 fasting. I put everyone on a Paleo diet. Most people will normalize their body weight on that. That takes a couple of weeks, but once they get over their addiction issues, they can do that. They have to drink good water. I want them to filter their shower and drinking water because that is one way to be exposed to a lot of junk.

I want to make sure they get enough sleep for them. Some people need seven hours. Some people need nine hours. I have another company called BodyHealth, and we make a sleep product that's really good. It's a natural product that helps develop natural sleep. They have to learn to get along with the toxic people in their environment or get away from them. It's like being a firefighter and walking into a toxic building. Very few people get better if they don't handle those people in their environment who are making them sick.

The other thing is that I don't think you can live in today's environment without nutritional supplementation, even if you eat good food and drink and bathe in good water. You need your body to be able to get supplements so that you can boost the nutrition in the body. We make a multivitamin that's on the market. It's called BodyHealth Complete + Detox. It's really good. I put everyone on that.

I give everyone amino acids because virtually everybody is deficient. We have a new product coming out called Perfect Amino, which is the best form of amino acids. Everyone has to take vitamin D. I put everyone on a juicing program or green powders because everyone needs that. Omega-3s and essential fatty acids are low in almost everyone unless they're eating a lot of fish. Those are my core nutrients. I tested 600 people for iodine levels, and 595 of them were low. You need to add iodine. Everyone is magnesium deficient, so you need to have magnesium.

Take those core supplements, eat a Paleo diet, sleep, manage stressors, and get exercise. Do something you like that's fun. It should be aerobic. Lift up rocks, turn tires over, or go to the gym. Work your muscles. If you don't work your muscles, they're going to atrophy. With that core program, a lot of people will feel better.

The other thing I do with every new patient is to give them a five-week course of IV vitamins, minerals, and ozone. Ozone is a universal gift. It makes everything better. We do ozone with the vitamin and mineral cocktail. They come in a couple of times a week. I've found in my experience that if I do the IV and the supplements, on a recheck visit in five weeks, 98 percent are well on their way to health. They feel it and they know it. Everything else after that is tweaking and tuning up what's unique for them.

. . . .

Dr. Kondrot: What are some key takeaway points on your approach or what are the most important action steps?

Dr. Minkoff: The thing that's most important is that your health is in your hands. Your genetics are usually not the big factor in why you can't feel the way you'd like to feel. My own genetic profile is not good. I have all the messed-up genetics you could get. My grandfather, mother, and father all had heart disease. They had heart attacks at young ages. I have a brother who had a quadruple bypass. I have another brother and sister who are way overweight and struggle with it.

By management of lifestyle, you can have control of your own health and make your own body healthy so that you don't fall in the hands of the regular medical system. If you do, the chances are that they will shorten your life. Medication for cholesterol, diabetes, high blood pressure, osteoporosis, and autoimmune disease is never a cure. It is only a Band-Aid. It's only a way to cover up the real cause of what's happening in your body.

That's why you need to take control of your diet and lifestyle and then find a doctor you can work with. It can be a naturopath, chiropractor, medical doctor, or nurse practitioner who is trained to see the body as a holistic unit. You can get better. The other part of this is to take care of your teeth. Brush your teeth at least twice a day and floss. Go to a natural dentist. Get your mouth healthy and it's not going to be detrimental to your overall health.

If you do these things, your own health can be maintained, and you can live a long time feeling really good. The ideal is to hit 120, and die of a heart attack in your sleep. Up to that point, you are good. When I was 40, I said, "What's my goal? I want to peak at 65 and then have 25 years of excellent health where I can be good." I'm in a peak of health for myself right now. Competition wise, I'm doing the best I've ever done. I feel good. I can work a full day, train for a triathlon, and enjoy my life, and I'm free of Medicare, medication, and any medical problem.

That's my goal for my patients, that they don't need me except as a guide so I can show them what to do and help them with the testing, so they know what they have to do. Then they can live a healthy life free from a toxic medical and dental system.

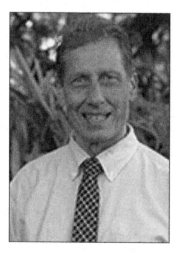

David Minkoff, MD
LifeWorks Wellness Center
301 Turner Street
Clearwater, FL 33756
727-466-6789.
Lifeworkswellnesscenter.com
Drminkoff.com
Drminkoff@bodyhealth.com

AN OSTEOPATHIC PHYSICIAN INTEGRATES MANUAL MEDICINE WITH CHELATION

Interview with
David P. Nebbeling, DO

Dr. Nebbeling was born in Holland, Michigan, and raised in East Lansing, Michigan. He completed his undergraduate degree at Michigan State University and graduated with a Bachelor of Science in Microbiology and Public Health. He then attended Michigan State University's College of Osteopathic Medicine. After graduating in 1986, he completed his hospital training at the Davenport Medical Center in Iowa.

Dr. Nebbeling has been on the cutting edge of alternative medicine for over 25 years. He lectures and assists with hands-on training to medical students, residents, and licensed physicians in the areas of prolotherapy, prolozone, chelation, neural therapy, mesotherapy, nutrition, and osteopathic manual medicine.

Dr. Nebbeling's current practice, Advanced Osteopathic Health, was established in 2005. He is also licensed to treat patients in three states, volunteers as a medical missionary, and is involved in numerous professional associations, including the International College of Integrative Medicine (ICIM). He is also regarded as one of the "Top 20 Alternative Doctors in America." Dr. Nebbeling is a father of six and an active member in his church and community in Lansing.

1. **The body is assailed by chemicals and heavy metals on a daily basis, and these toxins accumulate and disrupt our hormones and endocrine system.**

2. **Neural therapy is a form of alternative medicine that involves injecting anesthetics into specific areas of the body in order to relieve a variety of medical conditions, including chronic pain.**

3. **When people have proper nutrition, their urine will contain more toxic metals than people who are deficient in vitamin C, zinc, or magnesium.**

. . . .

Dr. Kondrot: Please tell us about your medical training and how you became interested in chelation and detoxification.

Dr. Nebbeling: I grew up in East Lansing, Michigan. Even as a child I was fascinated by medicine, so after high school I decided to pursue my dream of becoming a physician. After completing my undergraduate degree at Michigan State University, I was accepted in MSU's College of Osteopathic Medicine.

After four years of medical school at MSU, I went on to complete standard general practitioner's training. It was during my internship at an osteopathic hospital in Davenport, Iowa, that I met Dr. Wilber Huls, a physician who came from a distinguished family of osteopaths. Their approach to alternative medicine was ahead of their time, as complementary medicine was not nearly as advanced or accepted as it is today.

I decided to join his practice mainly out of my interest in osteopathic manual medicine. He and his father were both experts in cranial manipulation which involves working with the bones of the skull and the cerebrospinal fluid. I was not only drawn to their obvious skill and expertise but also to their impressive history of successful treatment and the healing they had accomplished in their clinic.

Interestingly enough, Dr. Huls' father, William Huls, was a good friend of another one of our mutual friends, Dr. Garry Gordon's father. Back in the 1940s and

1950s, Dr. Gordon and Dr. Huls were part of a revolutionary group of open-minded and innovative doctors. Some say that Dr. Huls' father was the first physician to inject ozone into the joints of patients.

When I first joined Dr. Huls' practice, my experience with chelation therapy was pretty limited, but I recall Dr. Huls assuring me that "this is something you might be interested in." He was close to retirement, so, although he wasn't personally responsible for my training, he recommended that I go to ACAM (American College for Advancement in Medicine) to complete my basic training.

While attending medical school and throughout my internship, the physicians I worked with knew little about chelation and most had a negative view of it. Before classes began at ACAM, they sent a packet of nearly ten pounds of paperwork and articles to prepare us for the training. As I studied the material, I remember being impressed with the amount of supporting evidence for chelation therapy and how it went along perfectly with the osteopathic philosophy.

Osteopathy is the American philosophy of medicine. One of the main principles of osteopathy is that God gave the body the ability to heal itself. The philosophy also maintains that the rule of the artery is supreme. This means that uninterrupted nerve flow and adequate blood flow will result in health and healing.

When I first observed chelation therapy in action, I viewed it only as a way to open blood vessels and improve oxygen delivery and nutrition. Of course, such results would help to naturally heal the body, so I saw no reason to question or oppose the treatment. I continued to research the treatment, and my findings led me to conclude that I should begin performing chelation therapy myself, or find a physician I could send my patients to. At that time, I focused on using chelation therapy primarily as a treatment for cardiovascular issues or to open up blood vessels. It was after I got more training that I realized it also helped with detoxification, or clearing heavy metals. These findings helped me appreciate the effectiveness of chelation for a variety of disorders.

. . . .

Dr. Kondrot: When you're trying to educate patients, how do you explain to them the importance of detoxification?

Dr. Nebbeling: I begin by explaining that I take a holistic approach to medicine, and that's why I evaluate their overall physical, mental, and emotional health before recommending a treatment. I go on to explain the importance of detoxification, as heavy metals are a common issue that prevents the body from functioning at its full potential. I explain that the body is assailed by chemicals and heavy metals on a daily basis to a far greater extent than people were generations ago. These toxins accumulate and disrupt our hormones and endocrine system. These pollutants are neurotoxins that promote free radical damage, which is why they are associated with cardiovascular disease, diabetes, and dementia. I go on to explain that the best way to begin treatment is with a heavy metal provocative challenge or a heavy metal mobilization test. This allows us to get an accurate measurement of the severity or prevalence of heavy metals in the patient's body.

Dr. Kondrot: Does cranial manipulation help to detoxify the body?

Dr. Nebbeling: Yes, it does. The cerebrospinal fluid is produced by ependymal cells in the center of the brain. Then it circulates around the brain and down the spinal cord. It is absorbed in the arachnoid bodies in the membrane that surrounds the brain. The interruption of the cerebral spinal fluid circulation affects the body's ability to regenerate, detoxify, and heal itself. Cranial manipulation also improves the lymphatic flow in the body. The lymph channels flow next to every vein, and they return the fluids to the body, helping move toxins from the interstitial tissues of the body. Along with other manual medicine techniques, cranial manipulation improves the lymphatic flow and greatly enhances the body's natural detoxification mechanisms.

Dr. Kondrot: What would be some symptoms that a patient might have if they had blockage of the cranial-sacral flow?

Dr. Nebbeling: A common symptom is brain fog. The patient may experience a lack of focus, poor memory, and reduced mental acuity. Balance issues are also common. Headaches can also indicate a blockage. In my experience, toxic headaches usually manifest as pain or discomfort at the top of the head, unlike tension headaches that affect the back of the skull.

Dr. Kondrot: Can you give an example of a patient who may have exhibited symptoms, and, after some treatment or manipulation, the problem was alleviated?

Dr. Nebbeling: I had a female patient in her late 40s come to my office with a list of problems including metallic taste, muscle pain and weakness, fatigue, headache, and arrhythmia. Her primary care physician was unable to relieve her symptoms, so she started looking into alternative treatments. She discovered that amalgam fillings are made of a mixture of metals and are over 50 percent mercury, which is an extremely toxic substance. After learning this information, she had her amalgam fillings removed, but not by a biologic dentist. Unfortunately, during the removal procedure, she was heavily exposed to mercury.

During my physical exam, I found no motion at the cranial bones and very restricted motion at the three diaphragms. In osteopathy, we consider the area around the first ribs and collarbones to be the thoracic diaphragm, the area of the diaphragmatic muscle to be the respiratory diaphragm, and the muscles and fascia of the lower pelvis to be the pelvic diaphragm.

I started this patient's treatment with a technique I use in my musculoskeletal cases. It is called neural therapy, and it involves the injection of preservative-free one percent lidocaine. I placed shallow injections around her skull to open up the cranial mechanism. I injected her tonsils and down the sides of her neck, over the carotid arteries, and along her clavicles. I did this to improve motion of the thoracic diaphragm and improve lymphatic flow. I then treated her with osteopathic manipulation and then performed a heavy metals mobilization test. The test revealed that she responded well to the treatments. She had improved motion and release of restrictions and experienced relief from all of her symptoms. The results of her heavy metal test showed her levels of mercury and lead were extremely elevated. In order to address these issues, I designed a chelation program that focused on mercury, and it included neural therapy over her liver and kidney areas to encourage blood flow and detoxification to those organs.

Dr. Kondrot: Please explain what neural therapy is and the type of injections you give. Where are they given?

Dr. Nebbeling: Neural therapy is a form of alternative medicine that was developed in Germany in the 1920s by doctors Walter and Ferdinand Huneke. This treatment involves injecting anesthetics into specific areas of the body in order to relieve a variety of medical conditions, including chronic pain. Neural therapy is based on the premise that any injury or infection that damages the autonomic nervous system will produce disturbances in the electrochemical function of tissues, or interference fields. Interference fields can result from injuries, surgery, dental procedures, vaccinations, tattoos, and more. These fields create abnormal electrical signals, or blockages, that interfere with your body's natural healing processes.

Neural therapy works to restore your body's natural healing mechanisms by correcting these disturbances and re-establishing your body's normal electrical functioning. The procedure involves a superficial injection of an anesthetic solution, usually lidocaine or procaine, into the interference field or other location. The appropriate point of injection varies from patient to patient, so in order to formulate a treatment plan, I obtain a detailed account of their traumatic events and thoroughly assess their symptoms. It is also important to consider the patient's individual medical history along with their symptom description and my own observations.

I have successfully treated a variety of ailments with neural therapy. My patients have reported relief from chronic pain, arthritis, allergies, burns, circulation problems, sports or muscle injuries, and more. This treatment also supports the detoxification process by increasing blood and lymphatic flow to the liver, kidneys, and other areas of the body. I highly recommend neural therapy and advise anyone who suffers from unresolved pain to consider this treatment. Overall, my experience with neural therapy has led me to conclude that it's an effective way to facilitate the detoxification process, relieve chronic pain, and alleviate a variety of medical conditions.

. . . .

Dr. Kondrot: What's really interesting about your approach to detoxification is that you believe in removing interferences using neural therapy or helping the cerebrospinal flow using cranial manipulation to help the body detoxify on its own without using chemical agents. Do you have any other techniques to help the body detoxify.

Dr. Nebbeling: When I go over the results of the heavy metal mobilization test with a patient and explain the treatment schedule for IV chelation, patients frequently ask if there are any additional things they can do to assist in the process of detoxification. One thing I advise my patients is to adopt an alkaline-friendly lifestyle. I explain this to patients this way: there are acid substances and alkaline substances. The relationship between acid and base is scientifically quantified on a scale of 1 to 14 known as pH. On that scale, 7 is neutral. Below 7 is acidic and above it is alkaline. The American diet is full of foods and beverages that increase the acidity of your blood, but you can help negate acid's negative effects on the body by balancing your diet with foods that promote alkalinity.

Furthermore, alkaline blood helps increase the effectiveness of chelation treatments by enabling chelators to bind more efficiently to heavy metals. I explain to my patients that a well-hydrated body helps maintain an alkaline state, so I recommend patients drink one-half of their body weight in ounces of water. I also recommend The Alkaline Way™, a technique I learned from Dr. Russell Jaffe who runs the PERQUE Company. It's an easy-to-follow method that is explained in a simple pamphlet. It involves a 100 percent reduced form of vitamin C that is provided through the company. This vitamin C is much more than the typical store bought vitamin. It contains potassium ascorbate, calcium ascorbate, magnesium ascorbate, and zinc ascorbate. This simple program helps your body maintain an alkaline environment. People who are low in essential minerals will retain more toxins on a daily basis than people who have adequate amounts of co-factors such as magnesium, zinc, and vitamin C. People who are acidic and who are not in a healthy alkaline state will accumulate more toxins every day. Individuals who are alkaline and in a good nutritional state will eliminate more toxins through their urine.

. . . .

Dr. Kondrot: When somebody undergoes a chelation or detoxification program under your guidance, what parameters do you use to measure the success of the program?

Dr. Nebbeling: I look at the signs and symptoms the patient first reported to me, such as brain fog, fatigue, and weakness. After completing chelation, I conduct several tests to evaluate the patient's symptoms and to see if there has been any significant improvement. One test I administer is the heavy metal mobilization test, which I repeat in order to determine heavy metal burden. I also perform an EKG to evaluate heart arrhythmia. For patients with atherosclerosis, I repeat an arterial elasticity measurement. Finally, I conduct a visual contrast sensitivity test to assess the heavy metal detox of the brain.

. . . .

Dr. Kondrot: Please give readers your takeaway points that you feel are very important for them to understand when it comes to detoxification.

Dr. Nebbeling: The thing patients have power over and that I have no power over is their diet and what they're putting into their bodies. In their home environment, they need to take the initiative to put in a water purification system and avoid foods which contain toxins. We're talking about more of a plant-based diet and a live raw food diet. We're talking about one that contains no GMO foods. That's a basic thing patients need to do. We're also talking about supplements. I have excellent ideas and training in nutrition, and I carry a variety of quality products at my office. However, the effectiveness of these supplements essentially depends on the patient. It's up to them to take the proper dosage at the correct time.

There have been several studies that have shown that when people have proper nutrition, their urine will contain more toxic metals than people who are deficient in vitamin C, zinc, or magnesium. It's important that they follow their physician-directed nutrition program.

The other thing is to stay in an alkaline state. As I mentioned, there's a very simple program available for patients. We make those products available to them, but they have to go home, calibrate their vitamin C levels, and maintain them. If they can maintain an alkaline state, they will be healthier patients. Everything in their body will work better, including their heavy metal detoxification or their chelation program. It will all work better.

Simple lifestyle changes like drinking pure water, eating healthy food, and keeping your body more alkaline can vastly improve your overall health. Everyone—regardless of age or health—should follow the steps I outlined above.

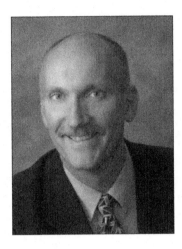

David Nebbeling, DO

3918 W. St. Joseph Hwy.

Lansing, MI 48917

517-323-1833

www.advancedosteopathichealth.com

OXIDATIVE THERAPIES AND CHELATION EQUAL POTENT DETOXIFICATION

Interview with
Robert Rowen, MD

Dr. Robert Rowen graduated Phi Beta Kappa from Johns Hopkins University, followed by medical school at the University of California at San Francisco. He has been board certified and recertified by the American Boards of Family Practice and Emergency Medicine. His philosophy is to assist the body to heal by providing what nature mandated for optimum performance and removing heavy metals and other toxins that inhibit health and healing. He believes that there are three fundamental causes of disease: malnutrition, toxins, and stress. Little in conventional chemical-based medicine addresses any of these. Dr. Rowen believes strongly in diet and lifestyle changes and promoting optimal body biochemistry.

He strongly believes that all healing ultimately comes from a Higher Source, but we must avail ourselves of what that Source placed in our world to assist our physical challenges. Dr. Rowen has been on a nationwide lecture circuit and invited worldwide to teach on oxidation medicine. He volunteers at a charitable Indian hospital, one of the few hospitals in the world open to integrative and natural modalities.

1. Forty years ago, we were told that DDT and certain pesticides were safe because we couldn't measure

them. We're finding out that even in parts per trillion these chemicals are poisoning the planet.

2. **People with brain fog, fatigue, and circulation problems started clearing up due to chelation therapy, and then we threw oxidation therapy into it. I'm absolutely convinced ozone and oxidation therapies help the body eliminate chemicals.**

3. **As we age and our bones turn over—more in women than men but in men as well—the lead comes out and poisons our organs and glands.**

. . . .

Dr. Kondrot: Please tell us a little bit about your medical training and how you became interested in chelation and other detoxification methods.

Dr. Rowen: I went to medical school at the University of California at San Francisco and graduated in 1975. I became board certified in family practice not too long after that, but I really never cared for allopathic medicine, having seen what I considered debauchery in medical school. I came to see that we were beginning to poison people with chemicals like we were poisoning the planet with environmental toxins. I almost quit at the end of my third year, but I stayed with it. I looked for ways to help people without giving them chemical medicine.

I first got involved in hypnosis therapy, then acupuncture therapy. In 1985, I was introduced to chelation therapy by a nurse who wanted to work with me because I was open-minded. We went to ACAM (American College for Advancement in Medicine) meetings together in the mid-1980s and started a practice in Anchorage, Alaska, that involved chelation and other complementary therapies.

One thing led to the other. I was on a roll with how to help people by giving them good nutrition, detoxifying metals and chemicals, and helping them reduce stress where possible, and get exercise. Then I got into oxidation therapy, and my life just exploded in this field.

. . . .

Dr. Kondrot: I wonder if you could share with us the most striking thing you noticed when you began to do chelation therapy.

Dr. Rowen: I had people who just didn't feel well. They had brain fog, fatigue, and circulation problems. These things started clearing up due to chelation therapy, and we threw oxidation therapy into it. I remember a man named Bill who couldn't walk more than 50 feet. After a series of chelation therapies, he was walking two to five miles a day in the Chugach Mountains in the backdrop of Anchorage. This was a stunning result.

. . . .

Dr. Kondrot: Chelation is still considered to be controversial, perhaps not in your mind or my mind, but there's still a certain amount of controversy. What advice do you have for the public?

Dr. Rowen: Consider this analogy. Forty years ago, we were told that DDT and certain pesticides were safe because we couldn't measure them. Now, 40 years later, we have the technology to measure in parts per trillion. We're finding out that, even in parts per trillion, these chemicals are destroying aquatic life. They're giving these animals mixed sex characteristics. Organisms may not even be able to reproduce at these low toxic levels that previously were considered safe.

Let's turn to medicine. Forty or fifty years ago, a safe blood level of lead might have been 40. Every year that goes by, it gets lowered. Now we know that anything higher than one part per million of lead in blood is toxic. Twenty years ago, this was considered perfectly safe.

Today, we know these levels are causing behavioral problems in children, circulation problems, and an increased risk of cancer. In fact, a researcher in Switzerland was doing chelation therapy, and he found that the risk of cancer plummeted in his patients. It was extraordinarily rare to see any cancers in the chelated patients.

Problems we see with metals today are real even though 40 years ago the doctors said, "It's impossible." We can actually measure it and see the connections. You have what's called the tomato effect where something that's out there really works and is real, but no one believes it. That's chelation. It's the tomato effect. (Editor's note: The tomato effect is a term used to describe popular ideas that are not founded on fact; for example, when the public believed tomatoes to be poisonous.)

· ·

Dr. Kondrot: You're probably most noted for your work with oxidative therapies, in particular ozone. I have to applaud you for your heroic mission to Sierra Leone to fight the deadly Ebola virus. I wonder if you could comment about the use of ozone in treating serious infections and your unique approach in combining ozone with chelation therapy.

Dr. Rowen: Ozone has been used in medicine since the First World War. They were using it then to disinfect wounds. Then they found that actually administering it had a multitude of wonderful effects. Since that time, incredible research from the work of Silvia Menéndez at the Ozone Research Center of Cuba, Velio Bocci of Italy, and others have shown the mechanisms of ozone. Ozone does several things. First, it improves the rheological properties of blood. "Rheological properties" means blood flow. The red cells receiving ozone therapy become more flexible. They can get through tight capillaries to deliver their payload of oxygen. The next thing is it actually improves the ability of red cells to release oxygen. Third, ozone modulates the immune system so that if you have an overactive immune system, it brings it down more toward parity. If it's underactive or not performing, it brings it up.

Ozone wipes out microorganisms, whether it's bacteria or viruses, in seconds. Chlorine is second best at 100 times weaker than ozone, so ozone becomes an ideal therapy for modulating the immune system and improving circulation. In fact, Bocci calls ozone's effect on red blood cells "creating super-gifted red cells."

What is the single function of red cells? It's to deliver oxygen. What is the most important factor in healing? Bar none, it's oxygen delivery. That's the bottom line in healing: getting oxygen delivered, burned, and consumed so your cells can make energy. Then they can repair.

· ·

Dr. Kondrot: Could you comment about the use of ozone in conjunction with chelation therapy and your experience with that?

Dr. Rowen: Ozone as a stand-alone treatment is phenomenal for vascular disease. If you give ozone, you can heal wounds, improve circulation, improve angina, and lower the need for blood pressure and heart medications. Ozone alone does this. I find that if you do ozone or oxidation in conjunction with chelation therapy, you speed up the process dramatically. I also found that I could probably reduce the amount of intravenous chelation I do if I use oxidation therapy with it. I may do less intravenous chelation and rely more on oral or rectal chelation while relying more on intravenous oxidation therapy.

. . . .

Dr. Kondrot: Many of the other authors in this book spoke about chelation removing heavy metals. Do you feel that ozone therapy can help mobilize heavy metals and reduce the heavy metal toxic load?

Dr. Rowen: A friend of mine who teaches ozone believes that ozone does chelate metals out. I have another take on it. Biochemically, it might be plausible. Ozone creates a lot of compounds in the blood called ozonides. They are molecules that are made from ozone's effects, and they're heavily laden with oxygen. We know that heavy metals are attracted to these oxygen molecules. For example, EDTA is ethylenediaminetetraacetic acid, and organic acids are loaded with oxygen, which grabs on to metals. Ozone may participate with this, and it may speed up the process. I don't have the exact biochemical mechanism. No one has really studied it. I think if we look at this, we would find that ozone and oxidation therapy combined assist the body in removing metals. Even if it doesn't do it biochemically, simply by improving the body's circulation, oxygenation, immune system, etc., you're going to encourage the body to eliminate some of the toxins. I'm absolutely convinced ozone and oxidation therapies help the body mobilize chemicals. We've seen it improve the health of a lot of people in Russia poisoned with pesticides. Chelation therapy specifically grabs metals.

. . . .

Dr. Kondrot: Can you discuss any other methods you use for detoxification?

Dr. Rowen: Detoxification is broad. We have metals as toxicants. We have poisons in our food as toxicants. Poisons also include food additives and preservatives, not only the hormones that are added or the pesticides that might be in there. There are so many different poisons, and our bodies are getting loaded with them. Now we have GMO, too. I ask my patients to eat organic, which dramatically reduces the poisons they're putting into their body. I suggest they consider saunas and sweats because that's a really good way to get rid of organic chemicals and heavy metals. It has been shown that sweat contains high concentrations of toxins. If you can sweat it out, it's a really good method.

We live in a really toxic world. The healthiest people are going to be using a combination of these methods to stay healthy. I myself went through intravenous chelation therapy. If I'm going to ask patients to do it, I should do it. I did. My heavy metal burden fell significantly. However, I remained rather high in mercury for a long time, so I put myself on my own oral mercury detox program, which I gave to literally thousands of patients in Alaska.

When I was in Alaska for 22 years, virtually everyone who walked in the door had five or more amalgams in their mouth, which automatically poisoned them with mercury. We measured them, and they were virtually all high in mercury. I was even high in mercury, though I only had four such fillings.

I developed a very simple protocol using simple, cheap nutrients, and it worked virtually every time. Fifty percent of the patients required three months, 25 percent required another three months, and I was in the last group requiring another three months of this. It was a slow detox, but my level of mercury came down from about 60 to 3, and it's remained there since. Yes, I'd like zero, but there's only so much I can do practically. I've had it checked periodically, and it hasn't gone up again. I no longer have any mercury fillings in my mouth, so I'm pleased with the results.

· ·

Dr. Kondrot: I wonder if you could share the protocol that you mentioned.

Dr. Rowen: It's very simple. I looked at what grabs mercury. Mercury is attracted to sulfur chelators more than it is to oxygen. Lead is grabbed by both oxygen and sulfur. Oxygen does very well and it's cheaper.

For mercury, I chose alpha lipoic acid, 300 milligrams per day. I used n-acetyl cysteine 500 milligrams three times a day, selenium 200 micrograms a day, and a couple of grams a day of vitamin C. All of these participate in glutathione metabolism, which is your body's principle detoxifier. Occasionally, I would add chlorella, sodium alginate, and sometimes DL-Methionine, maybe 100 milligrams. For chlorella, just take as much as you want because it's really a food. Sodium alginate is available as supplements. It comes from the sea and helps grab metals in your gut. You can also get metal binders and take them in your gut. There are a lot of things one can take that remain in the intestinal tract and attract heavy metals. For mercury, the items I told you seem to do extraordinarily well. It's slow and cheap.

You can also use DMSA, which is a bit more expensive. I think it's available even as a nutritional supplement. Then there's the more expensive DMPS, which is very active in grabbing mercury, but I think it has some problems. I've only used DMPS to assess someone for heavy metal toxicity. I never used it to treat them because I thought if you used too much, it could cause problems because it could take out some really good nutritional minerals. The protocol I described to you didn't seem to do that very much. I always have my patients take a trace mineral supplement anyway, even on the simple and slow method.

. . . .

Dr. Kondrot: Can you tell us about your method of evaluating patients for heavy metals and following them to make sure the treatment is successful?

Dr. Rowen: I suspect heavy metals in almost everyone. If you walk in the door, you're more than likely to have a heavy metal collection. I believe that you have to challenge—test—someone to see how much metal is in them. There might be better tests than this, but the simplest, most efficient method is to use DMPS, which is a chelating agent. In the past, I gave it intravenously to hundreds if not thousands of people, and I didn't have a problem with a single one. When I came to California, I realized DMPS was at least 60 percent if not 70 percent absorbed. Then we shifted the protocol to taking DMPS orally. The collection process is this: first, you urinate; then you take DMPS and collect your urine for about six hours because DMPS is eliminated quickly. Then we send it off to a lab for measuring, and we see what metals have come out. If significant amounts of mercury or lead come out, I can reasonably conclude this person has these metals. There are cases where I'm sure they have mercury and it doesn't come out. I believe that's because their body is not good at excreting, or it's tightly binding it. We may have to do this test again. Sometimes it takes two or three times to see it. This doesn't happen very often.

Chris Shade is a researcher who has developed his own method for mercury analysis using blood, which I happen to like. It's even more refined, but it's a bit more expensive. For the overwhelming majority of patients, the method I just described is going to be the most cost-effective.

· ·

Dr. Kondrot: Can you give an example of a patient you treated to illustrate the problems that heavy metals can cause in the body and the necessity of removing them?

Dr. Rowen: In Alaska, I worked very closely with three biologically minded dentists. A woman named Brenda was sent to me in a wheelchair by one dentist. She was in a total fog and absolutely dysfunctional. She could barely walk, and the dentist wanted me to work her up because he was scared to do anything with her, even though he knew she needed her amalgams removed. She had mercury fillings in every tooth. I worked with her with oxidation. I put her on my detox program before he did anything to her. She got well enough to have her fillings removed. Within a few months, she was virtually normal.

· ·

Dr. Kondrot: What recommendation can you give to patients for things they can do right now to improve their health?

Dr. Rowen: My mantra is that the pathway to healing is to deal with nutrition and toxins and reduce stress. For nutrition, this is my slogan. If God didn't make it, don't eat it, end of story. God didn't make synthetic, man-made chemicals. We did. God didn't make the hormones we're dumping into food. We did. He made the hormones, but they were to stay in the body, not to extract from the body or make in a test tube and put into animals. God didn't make GMO food. We did. Food was supposed to be grown in rich, organic soil. It's not. It's grown in depleted soil, so we've lost a good bit of our minerals. I think mineral deficiency is rampant in our population. Nutrition is first.

Then there are toxins. If you eat organic, you will reduce but not eliminate your toxins because toxins are everywhere. I believe people should sauna or sweat. I like the use of oxidation or ozone therapy. I recommend that my patients get an ozone generator. I like the one from Longevity Resources in Canada because it's reasonably cost-effective. I give a protocol to use for rectal administration. I advocate chelation, whether it's oral, rectal, or IV, depending upon your budget and the need to pull out heavy metals.

Exercise is very important. Every study out there shows that some type of exercise is crucial. Just routinely getting out there a couple of times a week to walk a couple of miles or hiking a few times a week and keeping your body active will help. Getting sunlight is important. We know we need vitamin D. In most of the United States in the wintertime, you just can't get enough. Even I supplement with vitamin D. Those are the basics.

. . . .

Dr. Kondrot: I understand that you're doing less in the way of EDTA chelation and more in the way of ozone. I wonder if you could discuss this.

Dr. Rowen: It's not that I'm doing less EDTA chelation. It's the way I'm doing it. I find that people only have so much money, and EDTA IV chelation is expensive for a lot of people. I've listened to my mentor, Garry Gordon, on this. He says that oral EDTA is absorbable. I've investigated this, and indeed it is. It's not absorbable like the gold standard intravenous, but even if only five percent gets absorbed, that's still far cheaper than intravenous chelation. I give my patients oral chelation with EDTA. Maybe it works slower, but they can take it over a longer period of time. It works.

There's also rectal chelation. There's a suppository that I've been able to get called Detoxamin. I can give it rectally, and it's at least a third to 40 percent absorbed compared to IV chelation, and it's still cheaper than IV chelation. Some people really swear by this.

Then there's IV chelation. I'm doing EDTA chelation. It is extraordinarily safe, and it's very effective, especially for lead. It also takes out cadmium and other minerals, but I was never super happy with it for mercury, though theoretically it should get mercury. Based on my own knowledge, I went more toward sulfur nutrients for chelating mercury rather than rely on EDTA.

Because of people's financial situation, I've done less intravenous EDTA. I've done more oral and rectal EDTA in the last five years. Then I used a patient's limited assets for oxidation therapy, which is clearly best given intravenously. Maybe they get a machine where they can do it rectally at home. I don't think that's as good as intravenous, but it does work.

Oral chelation does work, and there are a lot of things you can take that help mop up toxins in the gut. Activated charcoal is incredible at detoxing chemicals. I think people should stay on activated charcoal long term because it stays in the gut and acts like a sponge absorbing the toxins. As the blood flows through the gut, the activated charcoal or other intestinal detoxifiers sit there absorbing it. Zeolites are also a means of absorbing heavy metals in the intestine. There are many ways to skin this cat depending upon a patient's financial needs. We healers need to be cognizant of what a patient can do.

· ·

Dr. Kondrot: The takeaway point is you really have to tailor a treatment program based on the available finances of your patients. They do need to do something, and they need to do it on a daily basis. Do you agree?

Dr. Rowen: I really do agree. We have about 1,000 times the amount of lead in our bones today as the bones of our pre-Colombian ancestors in South America before the white man came and we had the industrial revolution. Why isn't anyone awakening to this? This is a calamity. The lead is stored in bones to protect our brain, eyes, heart, and circulation. Then as we age and our bones turn over—more in women than men, but in men as well—the lead comes out and poisons our organs and glands, if it hasn't already poisoned them earlier. This is a no-brainer to me.

I was called a quack in Alaska by noted cardiologists. They asked, "Why are you leaving a good career in emergency medicine to become a quack in chelation?" I said, "Because it works, whether you believe it or not." They ridiculed me. Now it actually has come out that chelation does work. There was a study reported in the *Journal of the American Medical Association*, which they had to notice because it was done to the most rigorous of scientific standards by a world-famous cardiologist. It was reported at the Heart Association's meeting, and everyone scowled at it. Why? Because of the tomato effect. Now it has finally been proven that it works, and they still won't believe it.

. . . .

Dr. Kondrot: Do you have final takeaway points for readers of this chapter?

Dr. Rowen: Everyone should be doing some form of detoxification and maybe combinations of detoxification because you cannot get away from toxins and poisons in our environment. The detoxification should include a detox for heavy metals and for chemicals.

I believe everyone should be eating organic food wherever possible. Follow the old Chinese wisdom, "Eat your food when in season, ripe and fresh." You do this to the extent that you can. We're not in the Garden of Eden anymore where the food was allegedly growing right out of fertile soil. The old Chinese wisdom is to eat food grown locally, in season, ripe and fresh, and on fresh soils. If you do that, you're going to be much healthier than if you don't.

The less you cook your food, the better. When you cook your food, you're doing something even the animals aren't stupid enough to do. I haven't seen a lion roast its meat. I'm not telling you to eat raw meat because then you'll die of dysentery from all the E coli that's in your meat from the processing. Just don't cook it to oblivion.

Don't eat fast, fried, refined, or processed food. This was never found on the planet before, and this is why people are dying from heart disease and cancer. This is the wisdom I have for you. This is the basis of everything I do and teach.

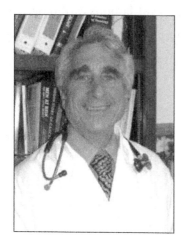

Robert Rowen, MD
2200 County Center Drive, Suite C
Santa Rosa, CA 95403
www.doctorrowen.com
707-578-7787

INTEGRATIVE MEDICINE CAN TURN YOUR LIFE AROUND

Interview with
Robban Sica, MD

For the last 30 years, Robban Sica, MD, has been passionate about integrative medicine, which is the synthesis of the best of conventional and alternative therapies, building a sustainable, patient-centered healthcare system focused on prevention and positive treatment outcomes. She practices integrative medicine with extensive training and experience in bio-identical hormone balancing, endocrine problems, environmental medicine, chelation/detoxification and IV therapies, nutrition, mind-body medicine, and many natural and alternative methods of testing and treatment. Dr. Sica is the founder, president, and medical director of an innovative and very successful integrative practice of natural and alternative medicine, the Center for the Healing Arts, PC in Orange, Connecticut. Dr. Sica and her affiliated clinical staff maintain a high standard of delivering truly integrative and preventive medicine and are dedicated to developing a new model for medical practice. Dr. Sica's practice has been based on the belief that health depends on the interplay of who we are and what we eat, drink, breathe, think, and feel. Increasing our awareness and choices about our health allows us to find a path to healing and growth. Active support, education, and empowerment foster the healing environment and assist our patients in moving forward on their journey toward a state of optimal wellness.

Growing a successful practice and helping her patients is only part of Dr. Sica's mission, however. Raising awareness about alternatives to conventional disease-oriented treatments with drugs and surgery has long been her passion, along with the desire to further cooperation and advancement of the integrative medicine and natural health community. This has prompted Dr. Sica to volunteer countless hours of time to a number of integrative, natural health organizations. She is President of the International College of Integrative Medicine, Secretary of the American Association for Health Freedom, and Vice President of the Connecticut Health Freedom Coalition. She was formerly the secretary of the American Board of Clinical Metal Toxicology and a member of the Board of Directors of the American College for Advancement in Medicine.

1. **Lead from the combustion of fuels that contained lead is still in the environment.**

2. **The new light bulbs are filled with mercury; if they break, you're exposed.**

3. **Chelation frees up the body's resources to cope with whatever other stressors the person has in his or her life.**

. . . .

Dr. Kondrot: Dr. Sica, please share a bit about your background, your medical training, and how you became interested in chelation and detox treatments.

Dr. Sica: From the beginning, I think I was atypical as a physician. When I applied to medical school, I was very interested in holistic health. At the time, I didn't realize it was politically incorrect to be holistic, integrative, or alternative. I actually wrote my essay for my application to medical school on holistic medicine. But my grades were good enough, and they accepted me anyway. I went to med school at what was then called the Medical College of Ohio. It's now part of the University of Toledo, so it's the University of Toledo Medical College. It was founded to train family practice physicians for rural Ohio, so I think they had a slightly broader point of view than some of the other schools I had applied to, so I chose to go there.

I wasn't particularly happy in medical school. I had a lot of thinking to do and a lot of wondering about which direction to go. I did a year and a half of internal medicine internship first. Then I decided to go into psychiatry, thinking I would get more understanding of the mind-body connection, psychosomatic medicine, and how stress affected health. Unfortunately, at that time, psychiatry was going through a huge transition from being psychotherapy-based to just prescribing medications, so I was not really satisfied with that part of my education either.

I decided to start taking courses in holistic health and medicine. I did a year-long training program in Boston through the Interface Foundation on different aspects of holistic health like hypnosis, various types of mind-body therapies like the Alexander Technique and the Rubenfeld Technique, Transactional Analysis, homeopathy, and a whole smattering of others. Once you cross that line and start to understand that there's a bigger world out there than what you learned in medical school, it's hard to go back.

I went into private practice in 1985, almost 30 years ago. I practiced integrative psychiatry at first, including psychotherapy but integrating nutrition. Back then, there were no integrative medicine programs you could attend, so it was a matter of learning different therapies and integrating them as I went along. In 1990, I took the American Academy of Environmental Medicine (AAEM) course, so I integrated environmental medicine and allergy treatment into my practice. I also took a lot of functional medicine courses. I started going to seminars, learning what I could, and trying to integrate it.

In 1989, a friend who was a chiropractor and nutritionist brought chelation therapy to my attention and gave me some of the old articles to read. I was blown away by the success of this treatment. I knew it was controversial, but part of me asked, "How can I not offer this to people who need it? It needs to be available to people with heart disease, angina, peripheral vascular disease, etc." I was so impressed by their research. I decided to train in it and start practicing chelation. In 1992, I took the American College for Advancement in Medicine (ACAM) chelation course. In 1996, I certified with the American Board of Chelation Therapy, which changed names in 2003 to the American Board of Clinical Metal Toxicology (ABCMT), and included more training on heavy metal toxicity. In 2004, I assisted in writing guidelines for a standard of care for clinical metal toxicology and chelation, by compiling much research and the work of other brilliant doctors, including Dr. Russell Jaffe, Dr. Jim Carter, Dr. Terry Chappell, and Dr. Ted Rozema. Three organizations voted to adopt that document as their white paper on chelation therapy and clinical metal toxicology, including AAEM, the International College of Integrative Medicine (ICIM), and ABCMT. I also recertified around that time in clinical metal toxicology with ABCMT. That's been my journey of doing chelation since 1989.

· ·

Dr. Kondrot: Your background is a little different from a lot of doctors. You began with an interest in alternative therapies. You didn't have that "aha" moment where your practice shifted. Please share with the readers what you feel the general public should know about chelation and detoxification.

Dr. Sica: Increasingly, we're being exposed to numbers of toxins in the environment, particularly heavy metals. Lead problems have been around for a long time. The background lead in the environment increased dramatically with leaded paint and leaded gasoline. Even though they took lead out of gasoline in '73, lead from the combustion of fuels that contained it is still in the environment.

A lot of us were alive back in 1973 and before, so we have a body burden from direct exposure as well. Lead persists in the body for such a long period of time and can have a profound impact on high blood pressure, kidney function, heart disease, cognitive function, neurological function, and memory. It can affect the mitochondria, so it can contribute to chronic fatigue syndrome.

Of course, there are other metals too. Even though there's been an effort to reduce mercury in the environment, we now have the new light bulbs that supposedly save more on electricity and produce less heat. But they're filled with mercury. Florescent bulbs are also filled with mercury. I think people aren't aware of that. They break one of those bulbs in their house, and they just clean it up and vacuum. They're actually dispersing that mercury through their environment, and they might not be aware that they're getting that exposure.

Many people still have silver amalgam mercury dental fillings which are 50 percent mercury. The longer they're in there, as you chew and drink hot liquids, the more mercury is released. It circulates around your body and gets into the brain and causes problems with neurologic function and memory. Mercury suppresses the immune system and has a broad range of other side effects.

Regarding cardiovascular function, mercury and arsenic have been proven to affect the cardiac muscle as well as increase the development of atherosclerosis. Heavy metals are a kind of a hidden secret. We all have some metals in our system, but most doctors don't understand or appreciate the health effects they cause. While these metals may not be enough to cause a condition by themselves, they certainly contribute to the development of chronic illnesses.

I always like to look at the total load of stressors and toxins in someone's system to see what we can reduce. From the point of view of heavy metals, it's always good to check and, if the level is reasonably high, reduce the body burden. That takes the stress off the immune system, vascular tree, kidneys, brain, and liver. It helps to free up the body overall to have more resources to cope with whatever other stressors the person has in his or her life.

As far as cardiovascular function and chelation therapy, I have had a number of cases that have been absolutely profound in patients' dramatic turnaround. Of course, all doctors who have been chelating for a long time have these amazing stories. In 1994, I got a phone call from a patient in the intensive care unit at Saint Raphael's, which is affiliated with Yale-New Haven Hospital. He was a 51-year-old diabetic who had had a heart attack in his early 40s. He had done maybe ten chelation treatments in a clinic in Mexico, but he didn't change his diet and he really wasn't doing anything else to help, so his heart disease got worse. He ended up having a pretty severe heart attack and lost most of the muscle in his left ventricle, so he had about a 20 percent ejection fraction. In other words, the pump was reduced by over two-thirds the normal pump function of the heart.

When I got the call from this patient, he was in congestive heart failure. The doctors gave him two weeks to live and wanted him to undergo a heart transplant because the heart muscle was so damaged. He didn't want to do that, so he called me from the ICU and said, "I'm going to sign out against medical advice. I want to come over to your office and get chelation therapy." I was a bit taken aback. I said, "I really don't think you should do that." He said, "I'll sign whatever releases and consent forms you want me to sign. I don't care. I'm not going to do this. I'd rather pass away in two weeks than go through a heart transplant." I said, "Okay. It's your body. It's your decision."

So he came to my office. We had to chelate very carefully at first. We gave him a lot of diuretics because his legs were swollen three times the size they should be. When he started out, he was short of breath if he walked across the room. By the end of 40 chelation treatments, he was walking 3.5 miles up and down hills, while he was on vacation.

He lived four and a half years. I believe he would have lived a lot longer, except his primary care physician put him on Rezulin for his diabetes. It's a drug which caused permanent liver failure, so it is no longer on the market. He didn't die from his heart disease; he ended up dying from the medication's side effects.

It was amazing. He lived four and a half years, and they had given him two weeks to live. That was one of my most dramatic cases and favorite patients. His wife would come in with him. While she was sitting in the waiting room, she was like the Walmart greeter. She would tell everybody who came in the door, "Dr. Sica saved my husband's life. This is what we're doing. You should be very happy you're here."

. . . .

Dr. Kondrot: If a patient comes to you for a routine consultation, what is your approach to evaluating them if heavy metals are involved and how do you determine which technique would be best for them?

Dr. Sica: I have an algorithm I learned many years ago from a holistic physician by the name of Walt Stoll from Kentucky. I call it the threshold. First, I look at the person's reserves in their system. In other words, do they have any deficiencies, whether it's hormonal, digestive enzymes, vitamins, minerals, or essential fatty acids? Then I assess what stressors are on the system, which could be emotional, mental, or social or stressors like environmental toxins, heavy metals, allergies, or chronic infections. I always want to assess all of those things, so I have a pretty extensive 11-page questionnaire. People are surprised by how long it is, but it helps me because I can quickly narrow down to what things are the most important to consider. I spend an hour with a new patient, going over their questionnaire, doing a thorough physical, and looking at all the symptoms they have. I pay attention to symptoms that point to heavy metals or a condition like heart disease or high blood pressure that would benefit from chelation therapy.

In our initial workup, we do a screening test for urinary porphyrins. It's a simple heavy metal screening test. If that comes up positive, even if their history doesn't necessarily point to heavy metals or vascular disease, I may suggest that we do a more extensive test for heavy metals. We also do an easy three-minute office test called the Max Pulse, which looks at the pulse wave to determine how healthy the vascular tree is and how distensible (dilation capacity) the aorta is. We can see whether this person is okay or if they are going in the wrong direction from a vascular point of view. It doesn't replace a stress test or other conventional tests, but it's a quick screening to see what's going on.

If they test positive in the screening for metals or if they have some disease like dementia, cardiovascular disease, chronic fatigue syndrome, or anything like that, I order a challenge or provoked heavy metal urine test in which we give chelating agents, which are substances that grab on to and pull heavy metals out of the body.

In my office, the patient is given calcium EDTA IV, followed by 1,500 milligrams of oral DMSA. Then I have them collect urine for six to nine hours and send a specimen to the lab. Many doctors use other chelating agents or protocols because there is no perfect way of assessing the body burden since we cannot directly chelate from many of the tissues in the body. This is an indirect way of assessing if this person has a large body burden of many metals or if they have the average levels you would see in the average person on this planet right now.

I compare it to raking leaves in the fall. We can rake up all the leaves that have fallen to the ground but we can't rake all the leaves that are still on the tree. So the urine measurement is an indirect measurement of what the body burden is. It's not truly the body burden because we can't do a biopsy of every tissue in the body to see what's there. It wouldn't be very practical, and the patients wouldn't be very happy with it either.

Depending on what heavy metals we find or what their other conditions are, I would either prescribe oral DMSA with glutathione or calcium EDTA IV to remove lead and cadmium. If they have cardiovascular or other conditions that would benefit from the longer chelation protocol, I'll recommend the ABCMT

(American Board of Clinical Metal Toxicology) protocol with magnesium disodium EDTA, which includes vitamins C and B.

For instance, if somebody has chronic fatigue syndrome, peripheral vascular disease, heart disease, dementia, or any of those conditions, I would consider the longer protocol. If they have scleroderma, rheumatoid arthritis, or other conditions that may be more related to heavy metals, I might recommend the shorter protocol because compliance is a bit better. Patients like it because it's half an hour instead of three hours of IV.

. . . .

Dr. Kondrot: One of the questions patients always ask is "How long am I going to have to do this protocol?" It is an investment, and sometimes it takes many months to a year before they're adequately chelated. What do you tell them?

Dr. Sica: I have some patients who just want to do chelation for prevention's sake. I tell them, "I would do 20 treatments. Then we're going to follow you every year and do another five to ten treatments each year."

If someone has severe vascular disease, I usually show them Dr. Chappell's wonderful meta-analysis study that he published in 1994 where they assessed patients' clinical symptom outcome after chelation treatments. At 30 treatments, 89 percent had moderate to significant improvement. At 40 chelation treatments, 91 percent had moderate to significant improvement. At 50 treatments, 95 percent had moderate to significant improvement. This analysis included studies of 27,000 patients, so it's a pretty significant study. I can then say, "Let's start with 30 and see how you're doing. I recommend doing it once or twice a week over a period of time. Try not to miss too many weeks." When they're done with the initial series, if they have significant vascular disease, I recommend maintenance treatments once a month so they maintain that improvement over time and their health doesn't decline again.

When you're treating heavy metals, the number of treatments really depends on which metals are present. Depending on how high the levels are, I'll start with 10 to 20 treatments and retest to see where we are. Lead is problematic because it persists in the bone for such a long time and that presents a whole constellation of issues. In that case, I might recommend oral DMSA with periodic IV chelation and retest every year just to make sure those lead levels aren't going back up from lead released from bone.

. . . .

Dr. Kondrot: Please share another chelation success story.

Dr. Sica: This is my own story. Chelation literally saved my life. Between 1990 and 1993, I started developing pretty severe chronic fatigue symptom, and I didn't know why. By 1993, I was almost completely disabled. I was working one to two days a week. I had a 20-minute commute. I couldn't even drive halfway without resting. I was going to bed at 8:30 p.m. to get up at 8:00 a.m. to go to work again. I had two small children. I was 30-something years old. I thought, "Is this how my life going to be?"

I knew about my mercury load because I'd had 11 silver fillings removed a few years before that, but at that time I didn't really understand that removing the sources was not enough. You have to remove the body burden of metal that's been released into your body.

In 1987, we had moved into an older yellow house, and we decided to have the old paint sandblasted off. The dust was everywhere, and it had lead and cadmium in it, and I must have absorbed a lot of it. So I actually had a triple heavy metal load. When you have one heavy metal, it has adverse effects on the body. When you have more than one, the bad effects are exponential. I was developing severe fatigue and exhaustion beyond belief, and nothing seemed to be working. It felt like I was encased in a suit of lead armor. Then I read a case report about chronic fatigue and chelation. Way back then, I didn't even understand the heavy metal connection, but I started chelating anyway. After I did the first chelation treatment, it felt like taking that armor off and I felt completely normal. After a few days, the heavy feeling came back again, and I had to do more chelation until finally my energy levels stayed high. I always say chelation saved my life. Otherwise, I probably would have been disabled completely for the rest of my life by heavy metal toxicity. While it's not always the cause of chronic fatigue syndrome, it's definitely one element that should be considered simply because of the way metals poison mitochondrial energy production.

Another patient I had a number of years ago was the mom of a chiropractor, who sent her to me. She had had a hemorrhagic stroke, but I'd never chelated anybody for a hemorrhagic stroke. I told him, "I can't guarantee anything. I don't know whether this is going to make a huge difference for her or not."

When you get bleeding into the brain, it leaves iron in the tissues. Iron is chelatable by EDTA. When we started, she was mostly in a wheelchair and could mobilize a little bit with a walker. She wasn't able to raise her arm above parallel to the ground. After five chelation treatments, she was able to raise her arm up to comb her own hair.

A couple of treatments later, she came in very excited. She had been using the walker to make and serve breakfast. That morning, when she went to clear the table, she just picked up the dishes, carried them over to the sink and put them down. Then she realized, "Oh my goodness. I didn't need my walker." She was ecstatic. That was after only eight treatments. We did a whole series, and she did very well. We were able to reverse the weakness from the stroke almost completely.

. . . .

Dr. Kondrot: What can patients do right now to help regain their health and eliminate their toxic burdens?

Dr. Sica: First of all, I would recommend they educate themselves about the power of chelation therapy. There are a number of good books they can read. They can schedule a consultation with a physician who's trained in integrative medicine to see if this may benefit them. Certainly if they are suffering from any of the diseases I mentioned or any chronic illness, they would benefit from a consultation with a good integrative physician.

My favorite organization is the International College of Integrative Medicine (ICIM). I was president for four years because I really believe in the mission of this organization. In addition, there are a lot of very good physicians who are trained through the American Academy of Environmental Medicine, the American College for Advancement in Medicine, or the American Board of Clinical Metal Toxicology. Those are other organizations where people can check for a physician in their area, since their websites list physicians and what services they provide in their practice.

I would highly recommend at least getting a consultation. You can always say, "I decided not to go through with this approach at this time," or "Let me see how things go." But just find out what alternatives you have, rather than taking medications that may or may not be getting to the real underlying causes of your health problems.

That's a concern I have about conventional medicine. I'm not anti-medication. Medications can be lifesaving. But when the only option given is to put someone on medication for the rest of his or her life and not deal with the underlying causes of why this person developed heart disease, dementia, kidney problems, liver problems, migraine headaches, or virtually any condition, I believe medicine is just not doing its job. It's always my goal to get to the underlying causes and reduce the dependence on medication or eliminate medication all together.

· ·

Dr. Kondrot: Do you have a closing story? Those of us who do chelation have so many. It's always gratifying when patients have gone through a lot of traditional care, surgery, and medicine, and finally a doctor comes along who really helps them.

Dr. Sica: One woman who came in a few years ago had really severe peripheral vascular disease. She was 58 but had no history of diabetes. Usually you see that condition in severe diabetics. She had had eight iliac and popliteal bypasses, and still ended up with an above-the-knee amputation on one leg. Her vascular surgeon said, "I don't know what to do to save your other leg." When I first saw her, her foot was completely white and cold, indicating very little blood supply. She had such severe pain in her leg and foot at night that she had to hang her leg over the side of the bed to get a little circulation there, which diminished the pain slightly and allowed her to get a little sleep. She couldn't use her prosthesis. She didn't have enough circulation in the intact leg to be able to walk with the prosthesis, so she was wheelchair-ridden. She was highly motivated to try chelation.

She did a series of 40 chelation treatments. By the end of the 40 treatments, her foot was pink. She had no more pain at night while sleeping. She was able to use her prosthesis, which allowed her to move out of a nursing type of facility into assisted living. She had an incredible improvement in her quality of life and independence. That was a huge success for this particular patient.

Another patient I had a couple of years ago came in with severe Reynaud's disease. The tips of her fingers were starting to die. They were essentially necrotic because of lack of circulation. One hand was worse than the other, but she was going to lose the tip of her index finger. You can imagine how painful that must have been. Her doctor was planning to do surgery because they weren't able to reverse it any other way. She started doing chelation therapy, and circulation was restored to her fingertips. She was completely out of pain after 30 chelation treatments.

In these cases, the stories are so dramatic because conventional medicine has done everything they can do, and they've given up on these patients. When you see a person's life turn around, it's very exciting.

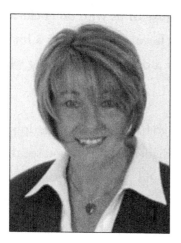

Robban A. Sica, MD
Center for the Healing Arts, PC
391 Boston Post Road
Orange, CT 06477
203-799-7733
www.centerhealingarts.com

ELIMINATE DEFICIENCIES, REMOVE TOXINS, AND TURN THE METABOLIC SWITCHES ON

Interview with
John Trowbridge MD, FACAM

John Trowbridge, MD, was educated at Stanford (Biological Sciences, with graduate courses in immunology, biochemistry, and pharmacology), Case Western Reserve (Medical), and the Florida Institute of Technology Medical Research Institute (Preventive Medicine). He received graduate training in general and urological surgery (San Francisco and University of Texas/Houston). He opened a general medical practice in Humble, Texas, in 1978. Since then, his post-graduate training has been extensive and expansive, and he is recognized internationally as an expert in several advanced anti-aging/longevity treatment strategies. Dr. Trowbridge has written several popular books and articles on The Yeast Syndrome, *toxic heavy metals and chronic illness, heart disease, and arthritis treatments. He has been recognized as a specialist in hormones and longevity medicine by the American Academy of Anti-Aging Medicine, in heavy metal toxicology by the American Board of Clinical Metal Toxicology, and in arthritis and pain medicine by the American Board of Biological Reconstructive Medicine.*

Dr. Trowbridge has lectured extensively in the United States and internationally and hosted radio programs on using drug and non-drug treatments for chronic and acute illnesses. He has served as president or director of several professional organizations, including the American Medical Student Association, the American College for Advancement in Medicine (recognized in 1991 as one of their earliest Fellows), the International College of Integrative Medicine, the American Board of Clinical Metal Toxicology, the International Academy of Biological Dentistry and Medicine, the American Preventive Medical Association, the NCR Research Institute, and the National Health Federation, among others. In 2005, his practice, Life Celebrating Health, was named one of the leading Centers for Advanced Medicine. His passion is finding solutions for chronic conditions that cause disability and discomfort that make life less worth living. Over the past 30 years, Dr. Trowbridge has developed and refined elegant hormonal, nutritional, metabolic, and other treatment programs that have resurrected the vitality, comfort, activity, and appearance of thousands of patients.

1. **Patients eliminate toxic metals three times faster by doing combination IV and oral chelation.**

2. **Chelation detoxifies, but it also rapidly rebuilds tissues and organs so they resume more normal function, including brain function. It's great when people can start thinking more clearly.**

3. **Chelation claims don't sound real because we're accustomed to organ specialists and organ-specific drugs. That's not the way this works. This works at the broad base of healing and repair.**

. . . .

Dr. Kondrot: Please tell us about your medical training and how you became interested in chelation and other detoxification methods.

Dr. Trowbridge: It's a simple, straightforward story. In high school, I decided I was going to be a famous heart surgeon since that was the era of Dr. Michael DeBakey. I got to college and decided that maybe I should go into medicine because you can think a lot more about medical problems.

I got into medical school and fell in love with surgery. I was training in urological surgery: kidneys and bladder. I realized that was a referral specialty, and I was far too opinionated (for many other doctors) about how patients should be managed, thanks to my background and training. I left the training halfway through in order to go into general practice.

Around this time, I managed to kill a fellow with Naprosyn, a relatively new arthritis drug that he had not had before. He did not tolerate the other arthritis pain medications. He loved the Naprosyn. It was fantastic until he bled to death in front of me in the intensive care unit, and we couldn't stabilize his blood pressure enough to get him into surgery.

I spent several months depressed about that and decided to accept an opportunity to go to the National Institute of Health. After my clerkship there, they offered me an opportunity to come back. I thought I'd go to law school or business school and do public policy medicine where I could kill people by the hundreds of thousands rather than individually.

At this time, I found out about laser acupuncture. We bought a laser, and it was spectacular in terms of the pain relief and other improvements we could achieve. I thought, "What else did they not teach me in medical school since acupuncture has only been around for a few thousand years?" I settled on nutrition as being the key thing I needed to know about. We had had four hours of training in my medical school. Rather than being an anti-doctor where you have anti-hypertensives, antihistamines, anti-arthritics, and so on, I found I could be a pro-doctor. I could promote health, so I got a master's in nutrition.

At the same time I was learning about nutrition, by chance, I talked with a doctor who had a busy chelation practice in California. He said, "Of course, you're doing chelation?" I said, "I would've heard more about that in my training or in the journals if it were a valuable therapy, so I'm hesitant." He said, "Come with me." He took me upstairs and said, "Here are my patients. Here are my charts. Here's my nurse. Have a great day." That blew my mind.

My dad had tried to interest me in learning about chelation a couple of years earlier because he was thinking about doing it because this doctor had recommended it. I said, "No, Dad. That's voodoo medicine." I was now eating crow.

From 1982 to 1983, I learned a lot about chelation. I took the preliminary exams and training and started taking care of people in the most dramatic, fundamental, wonderful way ever. Chelation is the crown jewel. That's how I got into it.

. . . .

Dr. Kondrot: What did you observe in the charts you were reviewing?

Dr. Trowbridge: There were two spectacular case categories. One was heart disease with people who were saying, "I no longer need to take my angina medication or my nitroglycerin. I have much more energy. I'm not short of breath. I'm returning to activities in my life." People with circulation problems were starting to talk about walking incredibly long distances. They were no longer limited, getting pains in their legs, or having cold feet. Those folks were absolutely real. I would talk with a patient, and then I would look at his chart. The difference between the parameters at the start of treatment and through the course of treatment was absolutely mind-blowing. I left there knowing I had to study this field of medicine.

I said, "This is the fountain of youth. Everyone is going to want this." That has not been true. A lot of people just want to go with the usual thing. Doctors don't want to learn about it because you have to go back to medical school and relearn your first and second years, which you promptly forgot when you got into clinical training. Chelation requires you to be a much more intellectual physician in order to get good results. Some do cookbook chelation where you use a standard approach for everyone. That, unfortunately, is available in quite a lot of places.

. . . .

Dr. Kondrot: You began as a non-believer. Then all of a sudden you had a shift in your paradigm. How do you convince people who should be getting chelation that they should investigate it?

Dr. Trowbridge: We encourage people to come in and talk to our patients while they're getting treatments. That's the exact same thing I did. People are very reluctant to do that. What we find fascinating is that our patients will be out there talking with their friends, neighbors, church members, and so on, and these people will see the improvements gradually occurring in our patients. Yet they will say, "I asked my doctor, and he said that wouldn't work for me," or "If only insurance would cover it, I would go ahead and do it." The answer is that's not true either.

The point is that people have to become fed up enough. They have to get sick and tired of being sick and tired in order to finally really look seriously at this. They don't look at it as prevention. They only look at it as a treatment, but it is much more powerful in maintaining good health than it is in restoring it. My job is to find the people who are interested in optimal health, who are already thinking about their future, and then show them how chelation fits in their program.

· ·

Dr. Kondrot: Do you have a unique approach to chelation?

Dr. Trowbridge: When I started studying chelation, I was intensely studying nutrition. The biochemistry of chelation intrigued me. What became apparent over time is that many of the explanations about how it works and what it does were simply wrong because we did not understand how the process really works. You have to remember this was the early 1980s.

What we have become certain of over the last 30 years is that chelation does one thing very well: it removes toxic metals from the body. Everyone wants to talk about how it improves circulation and this and that. What it really does is take out toxic metals. A detoxified body knows how to work better if the blockers are out of the way, and toxic metals block all sorts of functions inside the body. The only way chelation helps is by getting toxic metals out of the way so your metabolism can proceed more normally. You can heal, repair, maintain, and optimize just by getting the toxic metals out of the way.

What we do, very simply, is emphasize that we want to see your toxic metal profile, so we have patients do a urinary challenge. We adapt the treatments they get to the pattern of toxic metals that were excreted in the urine.

In 1993, I proposed a way of combining oral chelators with the IV treatment program. Over the last 21 years, we have refined that quite dramatically and shown that we get incredible improvements in reducing the body burden of toxic metals in virtually everyone treated with this protocol. We know we're on the right track because, as we reduce those body burdens, patients improve dramatically. Their symptoms resolve. Their condition gets better, their tissues work better, and they resume activities. That's the fun part. We get people out of their pain and on with their lives. We have very intense monitoring throughout the process.

Dr. Kondrot: Please describe this combination program using intravenous and oral chelation, and how you fine-tune it depending on which metal is elevated.

Dr. Trowbridge: We like to do a challenged urine test. We use D-penicillamine. The protocol is very simple. You take the tablets and then collect the urine. We send it off to the lab and get back your toxic metal profile. We also get an early hint about how well your nutritional status is with various normal minerals that are also excreted. That way we get a head start on knowing whether we have to provide additional supplements. We start doing the IV treatments. Generally, by the time the patients have had six treatments here, which is when we repeat the toxic metal profile, we say, "We're going to add some oral chelators to your program."

We confirm that at the sixth treatment and get another urine test. That generally shows us a lot more toxic metals coming out in the same pattern. If we're dealing with lead, we want to make sure we're giving the patient DMSA, which is a nice, smooth lead chelator. If we're dealing with mercury, we want to make sure we get them onto an oral DMPS program. If we're dealing with arsenic, we want to make sure we have them on a D-penicillamine program.

The patients don't take these on a continuing basis; we rotate them based on the metal pattern. They'll be doing D-penicillamine for a week, DMSA for a week, perhaps the DMPS for a week, and then starting over. A treatment program for rheumatoid arthritis, for instance, would be D-penicillamine taken through the day for several weeks, take a break, and then do it again. We are pulling out different metals from different tissues because the chelators work slightly differently. The oral program makes those metals much more available for the IV chelations which are going on, on a weekly or every-other-week basis in addition to the oral program. We're getting these metals freed up so they can easily be taken out, generally through the kidneys. It works wonderfully.

Dr. Kondrot: In your experience, how many IV sessions does the average patient need?

Dr. Trowbridge: That's a great question. Everyone wants to be done yesterday and have just half a dozen treatments. That's just not the way our toxic accumulation and release work. Toxic metals go in quickly but come out slowly. Depending on the patient's past exposure, we often see buildups of very particular element patterns. If they were closer to a smelter, they could have higher lead. What we tell patients is "We don't know how many treatments you will need. There are two things we're going to measure. The first is how your toxic metal pattern changes over time. As we see levels coming down, we know we're winning. We're never going to get all the toxic metals out, but we don't have to rush when we know we're winning. The second thing is your symptoms. Are the things you're concerned about getting better? Are you better enough that we can reduce your medications? Are you better enough that you're increasing your activities?

We tell them it's a joint discussion between the two of us about how they're feeling and about how the toxic metal pattern is reducing. Often the sicker patients will start once or twice a week, and we want to move them to every other week as they're clearly improving. Then it's every third week and then every fourth week. We call that a maintenance program. Our average number of treatments is somewhere between two dozen and three dozen. We are always moving patients toward a maintenance program, depending on their symptoms and their toxic metal pattern.

Patients ask, "How long do I have to do it?" We say, "As long as you want to maintain the benefits of reducing the toxic metals inside you. Remember that the nursing home costs $5,000 to $6,000 a month. Compare that to chelation, which is a bargain. You'll have years of healthier, independent, happier, comfortable living if you do chelation for a long period of time and keep taking out toxic metals that the environment keeps shoving in. They come in the air, water, and food. Since we're still going to live in this environment, we know it's ideal to keep doing the chelation.

. . . .

Dr. Kondrot: Since you added the oral agent with the IV, do you think you're speeding up the process and reducing the number of IV treatments?

Dr. Trowbridge: We actually tested that. From '93 to '95, I was trying them with one agent at a time and the IVs. From '95 to '97, I had figured out how I wanted to combine the oral chelators and the IVs. We basically had a three times faster reduction in the toxic metal patterns by doing the combination. In '97, I said, "From now on, everyone is going to be offered the oral chelators in addition to IV because the system reduces symptoms and toxic metal burden faster." Patients feel good, and we do it smoothly and gently so we're not putting any strain on the body's systems, especially the kidneys. People just get better and better. That means we can move them toward a maintenance program more quickly, which is a whole lot easier and a whole lot less expensive.

For those who are impatient, I tell them the half-life of the platelets is ten days. That means that if you have one million platelets today, half of those will be brand-new in ten days, and you'll still be dealing with the 500,000 you have today. Platelets are important because they're the blood components that get sticky and may give you temporary plugs that we call a TIA, a stroke that comes and goes, or a little heart attack that passes quickly. It starts but doesn't go on. Sticky platelets cause these early symptoms.

If you keep your platelets quieter and calm down the linings inside the blood vessels, you have a dramatically better outcome. I tell patients, "If you want to do it every two weeks, that's great. Then we're not just treating the toxic metals. We're using that approach to quiet down the process by which you might get very sick suddenly."

. . . .

Dr. Kondrot: One of the concerns with chelation is that as you remove these heavy metals, you'll have a toxic reaction. Another concern is that you may lose some essential minerals. How do you address these concerns?

Dr. Trowbridge: There are several different ways. Our chelation mix is very complicated. Around the country, the one- or two-day training programs say, "You need to put these five or six things in the IV bottle and give them this multivitamin." Our IV bottle has about 25 different things in it. Every sixth treatment, we use desferrioxamine, which is another chelator. We give them a vitamin-intensive pack that replaces vitamins and minerals. In addition, we take a look at the patient's condition, their medication use, and their ability to handle the stresses of their lives. We construct a personalized nutritional program for everyone so that we're providing the additional support, which makes it possible for us to use the chelators as well. There is a chelation stress. We are pulling out metals that aren't just toxic but are normal ones as well. We replace more than enough for the patient to gain health rather than stay even or lose ground.

The problem with removing toxic metals is if you try to do it hard and fast, it's a big stress on the body, so we do it slow and steady. We do very sophisticated tests to tell what levels are present and whether we're keeping up. A key thing in this is looking at their digestion. Most of the people who come to see us have some sort of digestive limitation. They've gotten older and things are wearing out, so they don't process their foods as well as they used to. That means they don't get the food value, which would include vitamins and minerals, from their food. We enhance their digestion and get that back into shape. We repair the processes that have been impaired, and people go on to do better and better.

Chelation is just a part of an integrative treatment program. It is the one that detoxifies, but it is also one that gives you the opportunity to rapidly rebuild tissues and organs, so they resume more normal function, including brain function, which is wonderful. It's great when people can start thinking better and more clearly. Their attitudes and moods change.

I don't know what kind of price I would be able to put on being able to wake up in the morning smiling and happy. That's what you do when you feel better. It's not what you do when you feel bad. Drugs don't do much to help you feel better. The chelation, nutrition, and fixing the rest of the body functions are ways to get a more robust and enjoyable life.

· ·

Dr. Kondrot: Can you give us some examples of patient transformations— patients who have gone through a chelation program?

Dr. Trowbridge: I can give you a great example of a fellow who had become very limited. He was in his 70s and had pretty much become a stay-at-home because it didn't feel good for him to get up and around. He had the aches and creaks of his joints. His muscles would cramp and were weak. He'd be out of breath; his heart would race, and so on. This was with the best of medical care.

I always tell patients, "You don't ever have to do chelation, but if that's the best they (conventional doctors) can do, I'd be thinking that something different had better be done." We started treating this guy, and, after about 18 treatments, he said, "I've gone back to work." I said, "That's a great idea." He said, "It's just a part-time job." He'd gone back to work at a grocery store. He said, "I'm doing things like stocking and helping with this, that, and the other." I said, "That's super." He asked, "Do you know why I did it?" I said, "Because you're feeling better?" He said, "Because I have to be able to pay you for these treatments."

He was just like so many other people. They have withdrawn from their lives. They have become reclusive because they don't feel good, and they don't have the energy to get up and go. Virtually everyone regains dramatically better energy. Of course, we're looking at the thyroid hormones, DHEA, pregnenolone, testosterone, and female hormones. We're rebalancing all of those as part of the integrative program because the whole body has to be reconditioned.

I look at chelation as a way of restoring the joy in life. It means a lot as you grow older to have your companions, your grandchildren, and your friends. People basically re-enter their lives. They become more social again. They go back to church when they've been avoiding it because they just didn't feel up to it. We celebrate our health and our lives by feeling good. That's what chelation does. It removes the toxic body burden. This is important. Never in the history of mankind have we had such a concentration of toxic metals in our bodies as we have now, and it's only getting worse. As you remove that toxic burden, you relieve the body of the strain, and it starts to function better because God gave us a self-repairing and self-healing body.

I tell patients, "We only do three things in this office, period. I don't care what your problem is when you come in." First, we find out what you're missing, if you need to supplement or change your diet. That's how you rebuild yourself. Second, we find what's blocking you from getting better. Generally, that's toxic metals, but it can be other things as well. It can be chemical exposures and so on. We want to get the blockers out of the way because that stops you from being able to heal and repair. Third, we want to find the switches that need to be turned on. Often those are hormones and such. We turn those on because if you throw all the stuff in the juicer but never hit the switch, you don't end up with juice. We want to turn on the switches at the same time we get the blockers out of the way and provide the raw materials. God does the rest. All we have to do is step back, get out of the way, and watch it happen.

Dr. Kondrot: What advice can you give patients right now to improve their health?

Dr. Trowbridge: That is so simple. First, drink more water. People just don't. They're walking around like camels. Drink more water. Second, get more sleep. We stay up late and get up early. We don't understand the impact that has on our lives because we gradually spiral downward. We are draining our reserves, and then we can't count on them because they're not there anymore. Third, eat more fresh, whole, raw foods, especially vegetables. After that, eat more vegetables. Beyond that, eat even more vegetables. That's where the liquor of life is. That's where your real minerals come from. That's where the health benefits of eating really come from.

Fourth, make sure you're getting enough oils. We tend to avoid oils because we think they cause fat. They don't. Sugars and starches cause body fat. Oils do not. We need to make sure we're getting flaxseed, safflower, sunflower, or one of the other good-quality oils. Eat olive oil. You need to get both sets of oils inside you. Then, of course, there are fish oils, the omega-3s. Then you want to eat regular meals. They don't have to be big. In fact, you can eat less more often. The more you eat three meals a day, the better your health. People who eat a couple of meals and then snack here and there aren't doing nearly as well as the folks who eat more regular meals and snack in between as they want. Don't eat so much. That's our real problem.

Get out and walk. At the very least, get exercise by walking because you keep everything lubricated and moving, especially the lymph fluid and your blood flow through all of your organs. That's a way of detoxifying your body quite well.

Beyond that, you need to start looking at nutritional support. The Department of Agriculture has shown that the foods we eat are deficient in providing the nutrition that they did previously. That's because in the old days, farmers actually grew real food. Now we grow agribusiness food. We have the business of selling food, so we want it big, so it weighs a lot and looks good. It doesn't need to have any nutritional content because it's going to sell if it looks big and appetizing. The kinds of things we are short on are vitamin C, magnesium, and the B vitamins. Those are very important. As you get older, you also want to make sure you're getting enough yogurt because calcium is extremely important in keeping good bone strength. Milk is not a good source of calcium, but yogurt is because of the way the bugs have predigested the milk.

. . . .

Dr. Kondrot: In addition to the good nutrition you mentioned, do you have some favorite nutritional products or a favorite product to help with detoxification?

Dr. Trowbridge: Two things that really help are sulfur-based foods. That would be garlic and onions. Those dramatically reduce the toxic burden inside your gut. There is a suggestion, though it's not been well studied, that when you eat those foods, you might be detoxifying your whole system. Other people are talking about using chlorella and other herbs like this to help detoxify. The other thing people miss a lot is that the cooked foods have lost a lot of their food value. What we encourage is juicing. Fresh, whole, raw juices are great. Vegetable juices are fantastic. If you need to add a little flavoring, add a wedge of lemon or apple.

We discourage a lot of sugars and starches because that's where you get the empty calories. The juices are where you get the robust vitamin and mineral content. If we can get people to do juicing, all that green helps to keep your body functioning better. It probably helps with detoxification too.

The one thing I offer as a final message is it doesn't matter what you have. If you're worried about lupus, arthritis, heart disease, dementia, or if your gut is a problem, it doesn't matter. We know that toxic metals are interfering in every system of your body. Just removing them will help that condition, often to the point of not having to take medications for it anymore.

One analogy I use is that every house has certain basic utilities. It has a road coming in and going out. It has electricity, light, and heat. It has food coming in and sewage going out. It has water coming in and trash going out. Those are all basic utilities. If you think of your house as a cell, then a collection of houses or cells would be like a neighborhood. That would be an organ inside your body. Every house in the neighborhood, or organ, has basic utilities. If you have a collection of neighborhoods, we call it a town or city. Those would be the various organs in your body, and every one of those needs to have all those basic utilities.

If you hamper one of the utilities, it doesn't just hurt this cell or organ, this neighborhood. It hurts all of the neighborhoods, and you start to see failing patterns in the weakest ones, the ones that have the greatest dependence upon that particular utility. That's where we start seeing disease patterns.

People think, "I'm going to see this specialist because he treats this organ, this neighborhood, inside me." What they miss is that all the other neighborhoods are also suffering because of the deficiencies in those utilities. They're either being blocked by toxins, deficient in the parts they need, or the switches haven't turned them on. When people think of specialist medicine, they think of organ-related specialists. That's totally wrong. You need to look at utility-associated specialties, someone who can figure out which parts of the cell metabolism need to be supported. When you support it in one area, you're also supporting it everywhere else. You're not just improving one system. You're improving all the systems.

If you remove toxics from one part of the body, you're removing them from all the others. All of them begin to function better, which is why there are all these claims about it improving this, helping that, and making something else better after chelation. It doesn't sound real because we're based on organ specialists and organ-specific drugs. That's not the way this works. This works at the broad base of healing and repair.

. . . .

Dr. Kondrot: That was an excellent explanation.

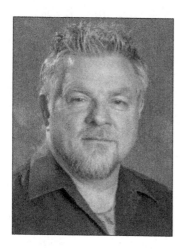

John Trowbridge, MD, FACAM
Life Celebrating Health
9816 Memorial Blvd, Suite 205
Humble, TX 77338
1-800-FIX-PAIN
drjohntrowbridge.com/

APPENDIX

Chelation Doctors Comment on the TACT Study

As you read this book, you will find many references to the TACT study. In some way we, the leaders and practitioners of chelation, are all thrilled that this study was funded, undertaken, completed, and showed chelation in such a favorable light. In other ways, we continue to be dismayed at the way the results have been reported. Still it is an unmistakable giant step toward establishing the credibility of chelation therapy. We look forward to the next few years as more studies are done and more great results found. Here is what happened:

In 2013, the federally funded TACT study was completed. TACT stands for Trial to Assess Chelation Therapy. Our tax dollars, $31 million worth, paid for a nine-year study to "determine the safety and effectiveness of ethylene diamine tetra-acetic (EDTA) chelation therapy in individuals with coronary artery disease." Could we reduce plaque in the arteries and other mineral deposits throughout the cardiovascular system in people 50 and older who had already experienced a heart attack? The answer astounded the medical establishment. *Yes, chelation can do that—plus other things.*

I believe the National Institutes of Health (NIH) agreed to initiate the TACT study because the medical minds at the table believed chelation would be proven a failure and that chelation would finally disappear from the scene.

The TACT study utilized 1,708 patients, 50 years or older, who had experienced a previous heart attack (myocardial infarction). Half received a placebo, half received the 40 infusions of chelation solution. It was double-blind, placebo-controlled—the gold standard of medical research. The way the study's conclusion was stated was based more on politics than medical facts:

Among stable patients with a history of MI, use of an intravenous chelation regimen with disodium EDTA, compared with placebo, modestly reduced the risk of adverse cardiovascular outcomes, many of which were revascularization procedures. These results provide evidence to guide further research but are not sufficient to support the routine use of chelation therapy for treatment of patients who have had an MI.[1]

Subsequent re-evaluation of the same data would tell a different story.

The lead researcher, Gervasio A. Lamas, MD, is a respected cardiologist and scientist who likes studying things and getting to the truth. Today, Dr. Lamas is unhappy with the official conclusions. At the time the study was finished and the conclusions were written, Dr. Lamas did not have the access to all the raw data. That goes to a third party—a company—with the idea the research team could be biased if they handled the raw data. The third party accesses the data and reports back "relevant information" to the research team. The raw data was released sometime later—well after everyone had read the *Journal of the American Medical Association's* (*JAMA*) report on the official findings and thought they knew all there was to know about the TACT study. That raw data includes things like the subjects' blood pressure, weight, kidney function, and all the blood tests.

Months after the *JAMA* report, Dr. Lamas finally got the raw data he had been requesting. He realized there was a much bigger story, and it had been kept from him. For one thing, the data showed a whopping 51 percent reduction in death in diabetics receiving the mere 40 sessions of chelation provided in the TACT study. Dr. Lamas has filed a grant application with NIH to do a second chelation therapy study, this one focused on diabetes.

The TACT trial showed a strong early benefit for diabetes and a weaker (or slower) benefit for the heart. Why? Experience tells me the kidney simply responds faster to dropping levels of lead than the heart. Had the test included more than 40 infusions, I believe the data on heart attack prevention would have been much stronger.

At the time of this writing, Dr. Lamas has submitted an application for a second TACT study and is recruiting enrolling sites—researchers who will then recruit and study patients.

---

1 Lamas GA, Christine Goert C, et al. Effect of Disodium EDTA Chelation Regimen on Cardiovascular Events in Patients With Previous Myocardial Infarction. *JAMA,* March 27, 2013, Vol. 309, No. 12

INDEX

*These chelating agents were mentioned
    too frequently in the book to be
    indexed. Their chemical names are
    given below:

DMPS
    2,3-dimercapto-1-propanesulfonic
    acid sodium
DMSA
    Dimercaptosuccinic acid
EDTA
    Ethylenediaminetetraacetic acid

CPSIA information can be obtained at www.ICGtesting.com
Printed in the USA
BVOW09s2307290315

393722BV00004B/11/P

9 781599 325712